LITE IS DANGEROUS

Henriette Chardak

LITE IS DANGEROUS
Investigating Aspartame and Other Sweeteners

Max Milo

Max Milo Editions, Paris, 2023
www.maxmilo.com
ISBN : 978-2-315-01140-7

FROM THE SAME AUTHOR

Shakespeare, l'espion des âmes, and *Shakespeare, l'œuvre au rouge*, éditions de l'Archipel, 2014.

Le songe de Baho la Chamane, with Henry de Lumley, éditions de l'Archipel, 2014.

Taül et les pierres de foudre, with Henry de Lumley, éditions de l'Archipel, 2014.

The Secret Passion of a Queen, Le Passeur éditeur, 2013.

Le mystère Rabelais, éditions du Rocher, 2011.

Cervantès : Plume du diable et ambassadeur de Dieu, Presses de la Renaissance, 2009.

Andreas Vesalius : Chirurgien des rois, preface by Jean-Didier Vincent, Presses de la Renaissance, 2008.

L'Énigme Pythagore, Presses de la Renaissance, 2007.

Dépossédée, Presses de la Renaissance, 2006.

Élisée Reclus : Un encyclopédiste infernal, L'Harmattan, 2006.

Kepler, le visionnaire de Prague, collection Les rêveurs du ciel, Presses de la Renaissance, 2004.

Tycho Brahe, l'homme au nez d'or, collection Les rêveurs du ciel, Presses de la Renaissance, 2004.

Élisée Reclus. L'homme qui aimait la Terre, éditions Stock, 1997.

Kepler, le chien des étoiles, Paris, Séguier, 1989.

PREFACE

It's about time! Finally, an in-depth and objective investigation of the ubiquity of aspartame in our food.

Aspartame is an artificial sweetener discovered in 1965. It is a dipeptide composed of two natural amino acids, L-aspartic acid and *L-phenylalanine, the latter in the form of* methyl *ester.*

Aspartame has a sweetening power about two hundred times that of sucrose and is authorized in many countries. It is referenced in the European Union by the code E951.

While it is known since 1983 that aspartame, very unstable in liquid form, transforms beyond 30 ° C in two toxic molecules, it is found in more than 6,000 products for human consumption (including drinks, pastilles, yoghurts ... and even in some drugs) or animal.

Used to replace sugar and thus reduce the caloric intake of food, i.e. to fight obesity, aspartame acts in fact quite differently! The consumption of products (drinks) sweetened with aspartame leads to hypoglycemia and prevents the feeling of satiety, causing a compulsive need to consume carbohydrates. Several studies have shown that sweetened foods are then absorbed in greater quantities, which leads to the appearance of excess weight.

Not only does this product "recommended" to prevent diabetes or obesity actually lead to a higher risk of developing these pathologies, but its consumption also carries other dangers.

The degradation products of aspartame (formaldehyde, diketopiperazine) are accused of being neurotoxic, mutagenic, carcinogenic and toxic for the fetus. Moreover, one of the constituents of aspartame, phenylalanine, is the cause in humans and animals of heart malformations and neurological toxicity in the fetus if consumed by the mother during pregnancy. A link is evoked with the increase in the frequency of autism spectrum disorders.

It seems therefore elementary to advise pregnant women to avoid aspartame during the whole pregnancy period. French members of parliament have been asking for a long time that at least a mention of risk for the pregnant woman, the fetus and the young child be added on any light product containing aspartame, but in vain.

The European authorities, including the European Food Safety Agency (EFSA), have never responded to this request. For EFSA, there are not enough studies establishing the toxicity of aspartame.

Moreover, according to EFSA, an acceptable daily intake (ADI) of 40 mg/kg/day constitutes adequate protection for the general population. Consumer exposure to aspartame is well below this ADI.

In May 2011, in view of various studies and under pressure from consumers, the European Commission invited EFSA to reassess the safety of aspartame and the validity of the ADI. Despite the publication of various studies, including that of Soffritti *et al.* in 2007, which warned of the carcinogenic risk of aspartame, EFSA considered that there was no reason to revise the ADI.

Once again, as in other dossiers, notably that of endocrine disruptors, the European authorities are more sensitive to the arguments of industrial lobbyists than to those of independent scientists.

In January 2015, despite the soothing words of EFSA, the French National Agency for Food, Environmental and Occupational Health Safety (ANSES) issued an opinion stating that no beneficial effect has been demonstrated to recommend regular consumption of intense sweeteners in adults and children. At the same time, it insists on the health risk of regular and prolonged consumption.

It is a first step towards the collective awareness of the damage that can cause aspartame!

Reading the book will make the consumer aware that the use of aspartame continues despite the risks it generates.

As is too often the case, the citizen has little choice and is invisibly forced to consume chemical substances whose safety is not guaranteed.

I therefore advise you to read this book carefully, because as Jean Rostand said, "the obligation to undergo gives us the right to know".

Corinne Charlier
Professor of Toxicology in Liège
Head of the Clinical Toxicology Department
Member of the Royal Academy of Medicine of Belgium

Introduction

Food is not food if it cannot feed.
If someone desires health, they must first be asked if they are willing
to remove the causes of their illness.
Hippocrates

I've never seen a skinny person drink Diet Coke.
Donald J. Trump, October 14, 2012

Aspartame is not a food but a chemical additive officially without risk. To prove its uselessness or the danger of consuming it, the investigation was long. The answers to my questions were often like a trickle of lukewarm water. Shrugs of the shoulders punctuated the thread of my curiosity. My file disappeared from my computer, so the safest thing was a hard copy, I resumed my investigation and changed the medium, but knowing that life expectancy was decreased for some people because of a sweetener did not touch many people in the so-called authorized circles to explain the facts. The silence bordered on denial.

It all started the day I quit smoking like a firefighter, by switching brands of cigarettes. I wanted to know why, so I simply called the manufacturer. Six years ago I was told: "We only put tobacco without additives in our cigarettes, that's why you smoke less.

- And that's why I have a cough?
- Yes, because we do not add aspartame.
- In other brands, there are?

- Most of the time the manufacturers add a cough suppressant. Before we used to put sugar, you know...

- But then if your cigarettes are only addictive to nicotine, you sell fewer cigarettes! What is your interest?

- We sell cigarettes to those who only want to smoke tobacco..."

Thus, I "foolishly" immersed myself in a strange backwards thriller, with some intimidation at the end. The result is a clarification on aspartame and its effects. This "sharing" book is built on four axes: the history of E951; the products that contain it; the sweeteners that are harmful to health; the citizen's response to an old political-scientific scandal that has remained in the shadow of the lobbies.

My book is for those who want information that is not obscure, not simplistic, or who are looking for the source of an illness that has no apparent cause for them or their loved ones.

Welcome to the backstage of world chemistry.

HISTORY

1 - FROM OLD SWEETENERS TO ASPARTAME: A MARKER OF TIME MADE IN THE USA

It is necessary to study all the facets of aspartame in order to understand the global health and food situation, because the history of aspartame is emblematic and sprawling. It is of the order of superfluous progress, even dangerous...

After hundreds of thousands of years of natural nutrition, uncooked, then cooked, cooked and seasoned and even gastronomic, Man has suddenly switched to industrial and chemical cooking. He hardly knows what he eats or drinks anymore. His taste buds are permanently fooled. From the privations of the Second World War to the exuberance of junk food, the sweet-tasting aspartame has become one of the answers to overweight. The progress wears several food masks for a so-called light nutrition but which weighs heavily on health. This is how the story of aspartame begins even before its discovery.

Saccharin, developed accidentally in 1879, was a phenomenal success before and during the World War II shortage. Soluble granules were manufactured in the United States by Monsanto. In 1953, cyclamate was added to cakes and drinks, which was ten times cheaper than using real sugar. In 1969, the FDA (Food Drug Administration) declared that saccharin could cause bladder tumors in laboratory rats, and consumers had to be warned about it by writing it in flyswatters on pink candy packages. Recognized as a carcinogen, good old saccharin went out of fashion at a time when people were eating high-calorie foods. In the midst of the soda boom, the market demanded a snow-white sugar substitute. Aspartame seemed to fall from the sky to support saccharin (still referred to as E954). It was also discovered accidentally at the G. D. Searle laboratory in Chicago. New prospects looked like a jackpot and a golden goose. In December 1965, one of the chemical engineers, James M. Schlatter[1] was working on a stomach ulcer drug, struggling to discover an inhibitor to the secretion of a gastrointestinal hormone. This detail indicates that the "worm" entered the fruit before marketing, because the hormone in question is the one that indicates to the brain the impression of satiety; restricting this hormone causes the opposite: appetite! As if in a scientific fairy tale, the mixture that had sprung from a test tube ended up on James Schlatter's fingers as a powder. He mechanically tasted the synthesized particles, white and acaloric: they had a sweet taste. The researcher had fortuitously recrystallized aspartame, but the molecule could not yet be infinitely replicated by the chemical, industrial, pharmaceutical and food industries. Before getting rich, the Searle laboratory had to prove the safety of its new product, which was suddenly non-medicinal!

In the spring of 1967, despite the sword of Damocles that is consumer protection, the future seemed bright for the old Searle laboratory created in 1888. It had just filed the patent for its "miracle" substance, and was preparing to carry out tests before the necessary approval by the FDA, for its dry use.

To start an internal study on the effects of aspartame, Searle chose the famous Dr. Harry A. Waisman, from the University of Wisconsin. In 1969, the expert tested aspartame in milk given to baby monkeys. In his experiment, out of eleven baby rhesus monkeys, one died, five others had very serious problems, heart attacks and epileptic seizures in particular. Waisman worked with integrity. His writings stated that the synthetic phenylalanine contained in the product could produce brain damage in young primates. He wanted to verify this by new research which started exactly on January 15, 1971. Unfortunately, at the age of 58, he died during a surgical operation. To be precise, and according to the doctor and nutritionist Janet Starr Hull, Waisman died in a car accident. The study was completed one month after his death. Searle submitted it

---

1. Research conducted with Drs. Robert Mazer, Arthur Goldkamp, and Patricia James.

to the FDA on October 10, 1972. All indications are that the results submitted were the opposite of Waisman's convictions as a researcher and pediatrician, a pioneer in the care of children suffering from a genetic disease called phenylketonuria[2]. As a biochemist, he had already banned phenylalanine (an amino acid found in proteins) in the diet of his young patients, ten years before the discovery of aspartame. He had described the risks in *Metabolic disorders and mental retardation due to amino acids*. But after his death, Searle "forgot" his analyses. Searle was then accused of having declared that the remains of baby monkeys could not be autopsied, preferring to submit another report on hamsters. The late researcher's independent view was countered by the US Department of Health Education and Welfare *on the* grounds of incomplete research. A new study was to be carried out over a period of 104 weeks, but it could not be continued because 30% of the test subjects died after 40 weeks. According to Searle, aspartame was not to blame. The zero-calorie market was on its way, waiting for the FDA to give the green light to sweeten a planet of coffees, desserts, candies, drinks and medicines. The commercial stakes were so high that they led to some of the denials that are still at the root of the media yo-yo phenomenon of FOR and AGAINST aspartame.

To impose a new product, it is necessary to provoke the confidence of health agencies and consumers. In December 1970, Searle developed a strategy to gain acceptance of its "sweetener recipe", in symbiosis with federal and congressional agencies. Old internal

---

2. Phenylketonuria has been known since 1934 thanks to the pugnacious Oslo doctor, Asbjørn Følling. This disease takes its name from the amino acid phenylalanine and from *uria* (elimination of a substance through the urine). There are 20 amino acids, and there is a rare genetic disease linked to one of them that causes a disorder in the metabolism of phenylalanine and is responsible for mental retardation. The livers of children with phenylketonuria no longer convert excess phenylalanine into tyrosine (tyrosine plays a fundamental role in the management of the body's physical and mental activity). Phenylpyruvic acid is a ketone. It is responsible for the characteristic smell and also for the name given to the disease. The famous Guthrie test allows to know if a newborn is affected by the disease. For the record, the amino acids are: alanine, arginine, asparagine, aspartate, cysteine, glutamate, glutamine, glycine, histidine, isoleucine, leucine, lysine, methionine, phenylalanine, proline, serine, threonine, tryptophan, tyrosine and valine.

memos show the art and the way to block aspartame's competitors. At a meeting at Searle, FDA officials were present. Excerpt:

"The basic philosophy of our approach to food and medicine is to try to get them to say, 'Yes.' To get things filed, we'll first ask if we agree on who we'd like to get a 'yes' from... We need to create a positive atmosphere. It would be nice if we could find people involved for these favors. It would also help put them in the subconscious mindset of participation."

To counteract doubt, it was necessary to provoke a form of belief. Aspartame would be the present and future "savior". Alexander Schmidt, the FDA commissioner from 1972 to 1976, believed that at first sight aspartame was a safe product, that amino acids could not harm anyone, especially in small quantities. We would have preferred that it was not "at first sight". Because as early as the spring of 1971, neurologist John Olney, one of the pioneers of glutamate and who had had it removed from baby food, told Searle that aspartame was creating holes in the brains of mice. A Searle researcher confirmed.

By February 1973, the company had already spent millions of dollars to prove the safety of its product. Searle delayed the release of aspartame to be "absolutely certain" that it was doing things right before marketing. A month later, one of Searle's researchers stated that there was no information to suggest that the product was toxic, that it was safe, but that further clinical testing would still be necessary...

In May 1973, Judge Turner, who had had glutamates removed from the market, met with representatives of Searle and members of the Chicago law firm of Sidley & Austin and discussed Dr. Olney's work.

In July 1974, the FDA accepted the restricted use of aspartame in food, but remained cautious about cooking.

In August 1974, James S. Turner[3] and John Olney opposed its release.

In 1975, Adrian Gross, a veterinarian at the FDA, wanted to make a new investigation on Searle's laboratory animals. He took up Dr.

---

3. Today, James S. Turner promotes stevia and is a consultant for Kraft Food, Quaker Oats, Hoffmann-Laroche, etc. He is a director of Swankin & Turner.

Waisman's work on phenylalanine toxicity. Richard Merrill, *Chief Counsel of the* FDA, asked the Chicago prosecutor, Samuel Skinner, to open a grand jury investigation. On December 5, 1975, Dr. John Olney and attorney James Turner waived their right to a hearing after the FDA and G. D. Searle Laboratory decided that the case should be heard. D. Searle Laboratory had decided to hold a public hearing, and because the FDA had put the approval of aspartame on hold due to the preliminary findings of its task force. Three days later, shareholders filed a class action lawsuit alleging that G. D. Searle had withheld information from the public about the nature and quality of the animal research in violation of the Securities and Exchange Act, an honorable action but one that carried little weight in the face of a desire to sell a product at any cost. At Senate hearings in January and April 1976, chaired by Democratic Senator Edward Kennedy, Chief Investigator Brodsky claimed that everything was "politicized" and that there was manipulation of information, but the *light was* soon to flood the market. In March 1976, however, the FDA asked for details on whether or not Searle's tests had been manipulated. The reporters of the investigation said that they had never seen such a badly designed test.

On January 10, 1977, the FDA requested a criminal investigation for falsified data. This was the first time the FDA had requested a criminal investigation of a manufacturer! On January 26, the Searle representative began negotiations with Judge Samuel Skinner, the *attorney* in charge of the investigation.

On March 8, one of the masterminds behind the Searle family business entered the scene: Donald Rumsfeld. Searle and Jannotta had offered him the presidency of the group. Rumsfeld immediately set to work in the heart of Washington.

In July 1977, David Kessler became the head of the FDA.

In August, the Bressler report was released. This veteran of the Second World War had compiled the various investigations of the FDA and indicated that out of 196 laboratory rats, 98 had died, that animals had been reported alive and then dead, noted again alive: totally surreal! Some autopsies had been performed one year after the death of the sacrificed animals. Errors were pointed out, confirming irregularities. Waisman's initial research was shelved.

Brodsky preferred to retire, saying, "The investigation gave the wrong answers to the wrong questions... They didn't even let the experts answer the questions."

G.D. Searle was finally able to invest \$19.7 million in a production facility. After Bressler's audit, Skinner, the Illinois judge, suddenly felt less invested...

On December 8, 1977, the investigation was dropped and the use of aspartame in food was maintained without restriction. When Dr. Betty Martini interviewed Jerome Bressler in 2002, Bressler told her about the corruption involved and reported that the FDA had made his file disappear! Dying in 2011, he had time to declare:

"When the FDA retyped my report, they censored it by more than 20% and removed the cover with the two mice that needed to be seen, and everything about excitotoxins[4]. You have to meet H. J. Roberts and Russell Blaylock to understand that aspartame kills."

Before continuing, it is necessary to understand what excito-toxicity is, a learned word that covers a reality: it is a pathological process of alteration and destruction of neurons by hyperactivation, via glutamic acid for example, or via all the neurotransmitter exciters that activate receptors, which in turn excite the neurons. This sounds complex, but our body is even more complex! But what do we find among the excitotoxins? Glutamates, NMDA (N-methyl-D-aspartate) and kainic acid (this one is present in algae and resembles glutamate, it is used as an anti-epileptic in medicine). In too great a concentration, this excitotoxic substance can attack cellular structures, which degrade up to the DNA... This mechanism is incriminated in a certain number of neurological and neurodegenerative diseases, such as amyotrophic lateral sclerosis, Parkinson's disease, strokes, Alzheimer's. Other pathologies such as hypoglycemia or status epilepticus can be observed. John Olney had noted retinal problems as early as 1969. But what remains of the debate concerning the phenomenon of excitotoxicity related to aspartame? The experts of the "pros" and "cons" are still arguing without agreeing.

---

4. Which excite the neurons until they die.

Before studying aspartame, one should have an idea that 40% of its composition is metabolized into aspartic acid: an excitotoxin. Since aspartame is rapidly absorbed, and unlike the aspartic acid contained in food proteins, E951 can cause peaks in aspartate concentration in blood plasma. Has this fake sugar that we absorb through thousands of products crossed the barriers of the authorities protecting our health without anyone being concerned? Yes, because the pressure of motivated experts resumed after the FDA's tantrum, a few bursts of morality cracked the citadel of the new fake sugar, and then justice chose an indolent slowness. Let's take a look at the chronology of this great blur... When Jimmy Carter dismissed Judge Samuel Skinner, William Conlon inherited the case. In January 1979, Conlon had joined the lawyers of Searle: Sidley & Austin, in Chicago, one of the oldest law firms in the world.

On July 1, 1979, the FDA requested an investigation into the manufacturer of NutraSweet.

On September 30, 1980, the conclusion of the report was *no approved pending, in* other words, no approval for marketing. Further investigations were requested, in particular on brain tumors. The conclusion was severe: "The (Searle) report did not present sufficient reasonable and certain evidence that aspartame is safe as a food additive.

It was back to square one. The E951 should never have been produced. But an election changed all that. Ronald Reagan, elected president, took Donald Rumsfeld on his team. Jere E. Goyan was fired from the FDA[5], and Arthur Hull Hayes Jr. became president. The aspartame drama was prolonged and an entirely new team of investigators was formed.

In May 1981, three of the six FDA scientists who had to deal with the famous brain tumors caused by aspartame, it was Dr. Robert Condon, Dr. Satya Dubey and Dr. Douglas Park who opposed the marketing of NutraSweet because the tests seemed to them to be unable to determine its safety. But Dr. Hayes rejected the results of his own team. In July 1981, he assured that the tests were favorable

---

5. His wife, Linda L. Hart, claims that Donald Rumsfeld said, "Goyan has to go," because her husband, Commissioner Goyan refused to approve aspartame.

and approved the marketing of NutraSweet. After this major, official turning point, Searle had high hopes for the use of aspartame in liquid products. The market would be gigantic.

In July 1983, the NSDA (National Soft Drink Association) urged the FDA to give its approval for the beverages. This seemed totally unthinkable because every good chemist knew that aspartame, which is very unstable in liquid form, transforms above 30°C into diketopiperazines (DCP or DKP) and formaldehyde, both known to be toxic. But the NSDA and the pharmaceutical laboratory Searle claimed again that it was 100% safe.

In August 1983, Consumer *Attorney* Turner and Dr. Woodrow Monte of the University of Arizona certified the contrary. General Foods[6] and NutraSweet had just formed a relationship. At the end of the year, the producers of diet sodas were allowed to sell drinks with aspartame. From then on, the consumer was informed as little as possible.

Between 1981 and 1983, the reign of aspartame began on shifting sands. In September 1983 Hayes received a flurry of conflicting reports at the FDA and in late 1984 the CDC (Center for Disease Control) began to investigate the first complaints from consumers who were suffering from symptoms possibly related to aspartame. It was necessary to evaluate the risk of induced diseases...

In 1985, the issue finally went to Congress. Senator Howard Metzenbaum, long opposed to aspartame, launched The Aspartame Safety Act. He wanted to alert the public and protect the 100 million American consumers. During the same year, Monsanto Corporation acquired the G. D. Searle Laboratory, while retaining William L. Searle, a former Army Chemical Corps officer.

Between 1983 and 1987, the American statistics of the National Cancer Institute revealed a 6% increase in the number of brain tumors, without being able to attribute a precise cause to them. With the arrival of new products, new unidentified risks have appeared. However, the boom in production and consumption always leaves

---

6. General Foods, an American company created in 1929 following the merger of several food companies, was present in France from 1963. A food subsidiary of Philip Morris, it merged with Kraft Foods in 1990, after the latter's takeover.

a delay between the announcement of health problems and the objective link made with their proven causes. In the food industry, a wave of "E" has swept through: E236 for formic acid, E621 for monosodium glutamate, E951 for aspartame, etc. The European Union authorizes 290 of them, not counting the 2,300 flavors that are not subject to any regulation. E951 was twice rejected and was looking for a world market, and it got it. Concerning NutraSweet, Robert B. Shapiro, the CEO of NutraSweet Company, told the *New York Times on* November 19, 1989: "Under pressure to try to expand the business quickly, we were rude, arrogant in an unconsidered way, we failed. We have changed." Shapiro went on to become one of Monsanto's top executives. The manufacturers always had time to turn around, defended by the famous law firm Sidley & Austin, whose clients included Monsanto Company and LG Life Sciences. Among its thousands of employees were two lawyers who would become famous: Michelle LaVaughn Robinson (marketing, intellectual property, transactions, etc.) and her intern, Barack Obama, who began working there in 1989. As for aspartame itself, the 1980s were rich in collusion and dealings.

In 1996, the American physician Ralph G. Walton denounced bribes paid by the aspartame industry to cover up the misdeeds of this sweetener.

In 2007, Bressler exercised his freedom to inform to finally get what he felt was not "confidential" released to the general public. The FDA's response came in 2008, signed by George F. Bailey, who made no apologies for deleting fundamental details about the toxicity of aspartame. Despite all the controversy and attempts at transparency, the marketing of aspartame was in fact a big business. Searle, Monsanto, Ajinomoto, linked to aspartame and the diet market, have always decided its future. This synthetic product has always been presented as a panacea, so much so that in the United States, sugary drinks have been banned in colleges and universities in favor of diet drinks. But is there a health benefit? Alexander Schmidt, the man who froze the approval of aspartame and ordered a commission of inquiry, Philip Brodsky, and many other investigators tackled a mountain that each time gave birth to a mouse, not even a laboratory mouse... The lie of omission caused sterile controversies.

1 - From old sweeteners to aspartame: a marker of time made in the USA

The lie of omission provoked sterile controversies, and consumption never stopped, despite the deception of the "merchandise". Updated in 2014, the official text[7] of the FDA concerning the approval of aspartame remains the same and specifies that it can be heated. Right off the bat, this is an admission of weakness from an institution that is supposed to protect consumers.

7. See Appendix 1.

2 - Collusions from the cradle of aspartame

The advantages of aspartame are primarily psychological in the imagination of consumers and many doctors so little trained in toxicology: a few hours on a full course! A cheap product to manufacture, E951 is found everywhere in mass sales and for the masses. No one has proven that it positively combats overweight and diabetes, on the contrary. However, it is found in more than 6,000 products: cans, bottles, lozenges, cigarettes, e-cigarettes, yoghurts, medicines.

Without the help of Donald Rumsfeld - the former Secretary of Defense - nothing would have happened so easily. Rumsfeld owes his fortune to *revolving doors*, an American way of opening doors between the private and public sectors. When he took over, the G. D. Searle was getting nowhere, until Attorney General Skinner resigned. Under Reagan, Hayes, the former Pentagon scientist, was appointed to the FDA and Rumsfeld boasted that he would make sure that aspartame was approved. It was. When Hayes resigned, he was hired by Searle's public relations firm. Sam Skinner, the "good" prosecutor, joined Searle's law firm, and later became Bush's senior chief of staff. He became a director of several pharmaceutical companies that privatize human assets[8] . The unbridled marketing of one side and the fragility of the "white knights" of the other have allowed the establishment of an underhanded corruption. The softness of corruptible experts and the docility of lawyers, who were

---

8. One of them is *Myriad Genetics*, which caused a scandal by filing patents on two human genes.

sometimes themselves scientific defectors, allowed laws to be tailored to promote a drug that had become an additive.

Monsanto bought Searle and then sold its share of aspartame to Ajinomoto. In reality, everyone remains a shareholder in one or the other partner, and the flagship sweetener changes its cache, like a game of hide-and-seek.

Chicago gathers almost all the protagonists of this thriller: the Searle laboratory and Donald Rumsfeld, who was born there, or Michelle Obama who was a lawyer there. In her "Let's Move" campaign to fight obesity, she poses behind a *"Monsanto Let's Move!"* desk. After using all her influence and popularity to fight obesity and creating an organic garden at the White House, she decided that children and students should drink diet instead of sugary drinks. Seeing her pose with Monsanto's blessing doesn't fit with her shopping manifesto, *Supermarket Shopping 101*, promoting organic and healthy foods. Her ambivalence made her applaud the use of aspartame for youth. Many American parents sent petitions to the FDA, not understanding that the First Lady of the United States would give a free ride to the soda industry filled with E951, Acesulfame-K, saccharin, neotame and sucralose. American scientists are still questioning her role and the way she has turned a deaf ear to the impact of diet foods on health.

Dr. Martini and Dr. Hum followed Michelle Obama in 2011 when she was speaking in Atlanta (home of Coca-Cola) about childhood obesity, unaware of Dr. H. J. Roberts' book, *Aspartame Disease: An Ignored Epidemic*. Dr. Roberts had sent his sister, Esther Roberts Sokol, to present the book to her. Security turned her away. Michelle Obama received a letter from the doctor explaining the correlation between diet and obesity. Dr. Roberts blamed NutraSweet, Equal and all *diet* sodas for their notorious effects on obesity, neurological diseases and psychiatric complications that he had encountered in his young patients. Was his experience going to change Mrs. Obama's mind as she had just used her influence to have diet drinks mandated in schools and universities? No. In 2012, then ranked as the eighth most influential woman, the first lady's opinion mattered. A *Juris Doctor*, she had previously worked for multinationals like Kraft Foods, PepsiCo, and Coca-Cola, But to be fair, after her *Let's Move!* anti-obesity campaigns, Michelle Obama advocated for drinking more water in her *Drink Up* campaign, promoted by Nestlé. In the White House, President Obama always drank a lot of *Diet Coke*. He would still drink it, as well as a former French president... Barack Obama especially protected Monsanto with the Monsanto Protection Act[9] of which Hillary Clinton was one of the lobbyists. It is a strange impression to see the cards of an industrial game that corrupts politicians: a global *House of Cards* where the players know each other and help each other without us knowing anything about it.

Dr. H. J. Roberts died on February 23, 2013. The man who sought to convince Michelle Obama that aspartame could cause confusion and memory loss, had also noticed the increase in Alzheimer's cases in some sort of correlation with the new biochemical data. He had developed a questionnaire so that everyone could find out their own reactivity to aspartame. Despite the legislative apathy, he did raise awareness of the right to health. But what could he change? After his 2008 election victory, Barack Obama put former Monsanto-types in key positions in federal agencies - those with power over food matters such as the USDA, the Department of Agriculture, or the FDA. Obama placed Roger Beachy, a biologist and former director of Monsanto's Danforth Center, in charge of the National Institute of Food and Agriculture. As for Michael Taylor, some of the American press mocked him, caricaturing him as follows:

"Hey, I'm Michael Taylor, former vice president of Monsanto, we poison everything you consume," followed by: "Hey, I'm Michael Taylor, FDA Commissioner, I'll protect you from assholes like me."

The warnings fell on deaf ears. Researchers blamed aspartame for an increase in autism cases[10] in the United States, to no avail. The "Monsantists" were the "knowers": Tom Vilsack, awarded by Monsanto for his activities in the biotech industry, Islam Siddiqui, a former Monsanto lobbyist turned agricultural trade and GMO export representative. At the head of USAID (United States Agency for International Development), Rajiv Shah, who previously worked

---

9. CBS source from March 28, 2013 (reporter Lindsey Boerma).

10. One in 45 children in 2014 in some states, double the number between 2011 and 2013.

in key positions for the Bill & Melinda Gates Foundation. And here, a brief "freeze frame" is necessary: the Gates are very big financiers of the Monsanto agricultural research[11], so much so that the couple owned 500,000 shares of the group in 2010. The powerful chemical industry has allies involved in humanitarian work. But Monsanto does not make cane sugar and does not sell non-GMO seeds... The Gates have a common friend with Obama: billionaire Warren Buffet, who took shares in the Coca-Cola Company in 1998. Buffett began buying 7% for over $1 billion. In 2006, he gave 83% of his fortune to the Gates Foundation and joined its board of directors. He can only be seen drinking Cherry Coke with vegetable extracts and no sweetener. On the trail of aspartame, we learn that the Gates are shareholders of Monsanto, and that Hillary Clinton worked for the Rose firm, as Monsanto's legal counsel. Obama appointed Elena Kagan to the U.S. Supreme Court. Kagan, a former deputy attorney general in charge of Supreme Court reporting, had already defended Monsanto in the Monsanto v. Geerston seeds case. Obama's biggest supporters, Bill Gates and George Soros, together bought 1,400,000 shares of Monsanto stock in 2010. The political world remains connected to the aspartame industry.

Senator Howard Metzenbaum described the FDA as the "handiwork" of the pharmaceutical industry: "The FDA's position is based solely on the Searle tests. Those tests are under a thick fog." According to the senator, G. D. Searle wanted the market at all costs, even to the point of swearing in the journal of the AMA (American Medical Association), that aspartame was good for almost everyone. His testimony in the Senate in 1985 resulted in a meager amendment: the legal daily amount of aspartame consumable. Thus, by 1985, lobbying and amnesia were alive and well in "blinding opacity", whether it was the Republicans or the Democrats in power. During the Clinton administration, the former vice-president of Monsanto, Michael Taylor, at the head of the FDA prevented any questioning.

---

11. Interview of Bill Gates on his GMO solution to fight hunger in Africa (GMO banana in Uganda) on the site bill-gates-gmo-farming-world-hunger-africa-poverty. Monsanto's GMO maize is already well established in South East Africa. With "Alliance for a green revolution in Africa" the African continent is now open to GMO seeds and chemicals sold by Monsanto, DuPont and Syngenta: names to remember.

And in February 2013, the Obama administration officially favored diet drinks with aspartame. With President Obama re-elected, an American article headlined, *"Obama Pushing Aspartame on School Children!"* In other words, the Obamas are forcing aspartame on schools. Could there be a link with Sidley & Austin? This firm, in addition to Monsanto Company[12] and LG Life Sciences, now advises large trusts. Ken Glazer, a specialist in anti-trust laws in Washington, after having advised Coca-Cola, worked at the firm. When Coca-Cola wanted to buy a Chinese fruit juice manufacturer (Huiyuan, with Danone as a partner), and was refused by the Chinese Ministry of Commerce, it was Coca-Cola's lawyers who reacted, all of whom were Sidley & Austin employees. Sidley & Austin is the best place to find out about the future of Monsanto and sweetener chemistry. Were the Obama's so nice couple so naive as to have wanted to impose light drinks that are saturated with it? By following the aspartame, we come across a permanent American conflict of interests between industry and politics with a surprising cast. To better understand on our scale, let's replace the American brands by French ones. We would all be astonished to see in business, not alumni of the ENA, but representatives of large trusts, and in majority of one...

- In the role of the Supreme Court Justice under G. W. Bush: Clarence Thomas, former Monsanto lawyer.

- In the role of the Secretary of Agriculture: Ann Veneman, a director of Monsanto's Calgene Corporation.

- In the role of Secretary of Defense: Donald Rumsfeld, a director of Monsanto's Searle Pharmaceuticals.

- In the role of the Secretary of Health: Tommy Thompson, who received $50,000 from Monsanto for his campaign for governor of Wisconsin, linked to Philip Morris, expert at Deloitte.

- Tied for first place: U.S. Congressional male hopeful in the contest for who received the most money from Monsanto: Larry Combest, well involved in the agricultural world, and Judge John Ashcroft.

---

12. Since April 11, 2007: Sidley & Austin LLP represents Monsanto in connection with BASF. They collaborate in the long term in the commercialization of biotechnologies. Bayer is in the ranks.

Let's not forget the supporting cast, and let's find a former interpreter of this tragic farce: Skinner, accuser and then defender of aspartame, director of operations for George Bush during the Gulf War, he had to defuse the scandal known as "Gulf War Syndrome", caused by the consumption of Diet Coke, which had been left out in the sun for weeks. Clinton made him his Secretary of Transportation, Clinton, who was particularly involved in the Searle and Monsanto court cases. In the meantime, the G.D. Searle Group has become a Pfizer company, which has been linked to Monsanto since 1997. But Monsanto has divested itself of the hot potato that is aspartame. The manufacturing is now done by Ajinomoto (40% of the market). Equal was sold to Meriant[13] which markets Canderel, and NutraSweet Company was sold to J. W. Childs. This man consults with Deloitte & Touche[14], which represents the interests of Kraft Foods and audits half of the CAC 40. While diet drinks and sweeteners change hands all the time, everything seems sealed in one circle. Bayer and Monsanto are partners, "married" or not, they have been "engaged" for a long time. As for the gullible consumers, they are sometimes transformed into guinea pigs who ignore themselves. They have light dispensers in their workplaces. They are offered dreams, or rather illusions. The Coca-Cola brand associated with the universal vector that is sport seems to promote health while sugar and aspartame cause addiction. Do diet drinkers think that an advertising slogan is worth the scientific truth and the precautionary principle? A real gap persists between noble and cynical industry, and the American law protects the business more than the consumer. But European laws are no better, the lock-in is practically the same.

---

13. Merisant holds more than a third of the low-calorie tabletop sweetener market.

14. Deloitte is a global leader in the so-called *Big Four*. Its revenues reached $28.8 billion in 2011. It is the largest auditing firm in the world, with 182,000 employees. A financial advisor, growth indicator, sponsorship and tax specialist, it is a firm, not a company. The group is now called Deloitte Touche Tohmatsu. Tohmatsu is also the advisor of Ajinomoto. Its network is grouped within a Swiss *verein* ("club" or "association"). In France, Deloitte is the leading audit firm since 2009. Deloitte reported worldwide revenue of $38.8 billion for the year ended May 31, 2017, representing annual growth of 7.1%.

3 - Consumption and issues for large groups

To digest all this information, avoid taking an Alka-Seltzer tablet, it contains aspartame. Which manufacturer does not use it? Everything that is advertised as sugar free, contains *sweeteners* most of the time. Ajinomoto, the market leader in aspartame, manufactures it, but the Japanese only consume the product made from stevia. Ajinomoto bought the license from Monsanto in 2000, and its earnings are in the billions of dollars. The giant Kellogg's has partnered with the Japanese giant Ajinomoto. Are they all unaware that aspartame and glutamate are true neurotoxic chameleons? They blend into a food landscape where no one is policing: "the papers are in order" in a well maintained legal blur. We can face the aspartame/glutamate duo in some morning cereals without knowing it and the *believers* in a magic product testify with an almost religious fervor on dedicated websites that all this is good for our health. And if they still get fat, they blame themselves and continue to consume diet products.

Is life good in Canderel? Yes, according to the European Food Safety Authority (EFSA), which considers aspartame safe even for pregnant women. The scaremongering is nothing more than a *hoax* written by the scaremongers or ill-intentioned sugar competitors. The lobbies are established at the EFSA and the marketing does the rest, it even adjusts to the commandments and religious precepts by Coke aspartame hallal and kosher. We find these treasures of adaptation on the Chinese site Alibaba, the largest global site for businesses, created by Jack Ma in 1999, also a retailer of Ajinomoto...

Religion or not, who does not want to refine his line or fight against diabetes if he suffers? If Canderel advises E951 to pregnant women, there would be no danger in the human home... Swallowing C14H18N2O5 - chemical formula of aspartame -, it would be as good as drinking spring water, hydrating and without risk?

At this stage of the investigation, we understand that aspartame appears in the media only as the tip of an iceberg. Doctors, patients, journalists, simple curious consumers, do not have a sufficient data base to think about the "benefit/risk" of using aspartame or other sweeteners for health. The stakes are high because aspartame is much cheaper to manufacture than real sugar. Not only does it mask certain tastes and whet the appetite, but it also stimulates the appetite of manufacturers...

Get your calculators ready... Knowing that a kilo of sugar was worth about 3 euros not long ago, and that a kilo of aspartame is sold for 12 to 15 euros per kilo but that it sugars two hundred times more and is three hundred times cheaper than sugar: calculate the profit margin of the sellers per ton of aspartame used.

Stevia is worth about 250 euros per kilo, so it is less profitable than aspartame. Since the FDA has approved aspartame for desserts, beverages and cooking, the "experts" encourage consumers to trust sweeteners, and even more powerful ones like neotame and advantame are available, without anyone being concerned. It is not only humans who consume aspartame.

On average, 850,000 tons per year are used for cattle feed. This is called white biotechnology. Craig Petray, the head of NutraSweet Company claimed that the sweetos substitute was saving farmers money. Sweetos makes a livestock *sweetener* and the patent belongs to NutraSweet Company. "We used to give molasses to factory-farmed animals, now we give neotame to mask some of the taste," says Mohan Nair, a health solutions specialist in Oregon, who says that sweetos[15] in powder, or liquid "is good for livestock who consume faster." The agricultural press confirms that cattle "get fat faster..." For the attention of lovers of these trough and table sweeteners, be aware

---

15. Manufacturing is often outsourced. The Indian partner who manufactures it is called EnSigns Health Care Pvt Ltd. You can easily buy it on the Internet for baking...

that the super-aspartame E961 is already present in our gullets as in Carrefour lime flavored cottage cheese at 0%. All over the world, we ingest products that are not innocent, but without our knowledge. They should make us lose weight, but they fatten the cattle. Curious this E961 developed by Monsanto: it is eight thousand times sweeter. And if there is an excess of consumption of harmful "E", neurological diseases will only be apparent when they are practically irreversible. If we look at the world of issues, we understand that consumption is not linked to health but to the profits of the food industry and pharmaceutical or veterinary laboratories. Discount supermarkets like aspartame only because it is profitable. Moreover, food manufacturers use it without always specifying it. In France, the Système U group seems to be the only one to have backed down regarding its own products without more aspartame. A website - openfoodfacts - gives the complete composition of the products.

Now we need to know who is making and using aspartame. Actually, it's a pretty logical puzzle... NutraSweet Company, one of Searle's divisions, is part of Monsanto linked to Ajinomoto and the global loop seems to be complete: manufacturers supply food megacorporations galore.

Nestlé is the leading group in sales volume in beverages (Nestea, Aquarel, Perrier). The slogan of the Swiss group is "*Good food, Good life*"; the group has bought the infant subsidiary of Pfizer (ex-Searle). In its Nestlé Health Science department, Nestlé has changed Dietsource to Sweet n'free and promotes aspartame in India more than in Europe. But Nestle Pure life Splash sold in the United States is guaranteed to be aspartame free. Would American consumers no longer be so willing to sell off stocks of E951?

Kraft Foods, an American group, is the world's number two food and beverage company. Until 2007, it was the Altria consortium, formerly called Philip Morris Corporation... and of course aspartame and acesulfame are found in cigarettes. Kraft Foods Europe has a myriad of well-known brands and their products are full of both additives. 80% of their confectionery is sugar-free, i.e. with sweeteners, some of which do not need to be reported.

Walmart is a giant of the distribution which weighs more than 400 billion and sells in its shelves 35 % of *soft drink* with aspartame.

Its British subsidiary is called ASDA, which refused to sell aspartame products. This made the Japanese manufacturer Ajinomoto mad, which, after a procedure before the British High Court, succeeded in prohibiting him not to sell aspartame.

General Mills, an American company and the world's sixth largest food group, has a portfolio of more than 100 brands, many of which are leaders in their markets and the French market. They are looking to replace aspartame with sucralose. Their Yoplait free is now aspartame free.

Danone, a French group and world leader in dairy products, launched its probiotic yogurts with stevia in 2006. But Danone also sells low-fat products, except for aspartame, and promotes them to endocrinologists.

All of these large global groups sell many flavored and sweetened waters with aspartame and acesulfame-K. These drinks keep the taste of sugar alive.

The Coca-Cola Company is one of the world's largest soft drink companies and its competitor is PepsiCo. Coca-Cola is known by 94% of the world's population and its *low-carb* beverages benefit from one of the biggest global advertisements. It is probably the best known brand in the world and uses aspartame extensively. In South American countries, the water used to make Coca-Cola is lacking, and young children are reduced to drinking regular or diet Coke. However, it is possible to become addicted to diet. In the UK, millions of pounds have been donated by Coca-Cola to British researchers fighting obesity and to the European Hydration Institute (EHI). Shell and Coca have partnered in a campaign to prevent drivers from becoming dehydrated while driving. The market is growing!

But what is in a *Diet Coke* for example? Caramel E150d with ammoniacal sulfite, bisphenol A, and E951. It is this same product, not nicotine, which makes smokers addicted. Professor Jean-Pol Tassin, neurobiologist and director of research at Inserm, has demonstrated this without any real echo. Would the food chemistry be a witch's apprentice? It only asks that the aspartame sodas are not left in the sun, that is why the consumer is asked to drink very fresh, without any other explanation. Small industrial groups do not escape aspartame. What does Ricola say about its famous herbal candy?

"We use aspartame because it offers a very balanced taste and is safe for teeth. We are convinced that aspartame is safe for your health, as evidenced by expert opinions and recommendations from internationally recognized organizations. Aspartame is probably the best studied sweetener, as it is used in a variety of products around the world. Independent international organizations such as the Joint FAO/WHO Expert Committee on Food Additives and the European Food Safety Authority (EFSA) have verified the safety of aspartame and confirmed that its consumption does not pose a risk to humans."

It could not be more reassuring. But these formatted and repeated phrases form a screen for criticism. "Let's stay calm", as the Nutrition Director of Coca-Cola France said. After studying in the United States and having served Danone, Coca-Cola Company, Mars/MasterFoods, Ms. Maha Tahiri, Director of Health and Nutrition for Bell Institute, is now working for General Mills (in joint venture with Nestlé) as Vice President. We could read her in an "advertorial" in the French press, attesting to the safety of the sweetener most used in the world. The nutrition director of Coca-Cola France was serene. To counter the undecideds, she talked about two brochures to explain the interest of diet drinks, one intended for doctors, the other for consumers. "We expose the positive role that light drinks can play in weight control. They contribute to hydration by providing the pleasure of sweetness, without the calories. "Sweetener consumers do not have a sweeter diet than others." Further on she claimed that "our brain is able to distinguish a sweetener from a sugar molecule." In October 2007, this doctorate holder in human nutrition was about to convince health professionals. When asked whether the brain can tell the difference between sugar and fake sugar, one thing is certain: both stimulate the reward circuits. The sensation of sugar makes the brain believe that there will be a pleasant energy intake. But without it, what about the desire for calories? The answer today is on the edulcorants.eu website: "replacing sugar with low-calorie sweeteners does not influence the feeling of hunger." This argument does not demonstrate anything and we remain hungry...

Pharmaceutical laboratories and manufacturers of aspartame products have the same private or state defenders. They all remain calm because the FDA has always defended the industry. One of its former commissioners, Dr. Herbert Ley, bravely stated, "The FDA protects Big Pharma and is subsequently rewarded for doing so, and, using the police powers of government, attacks those who threaten Big Pharma. People think the FDA protects them. It doesn't. What the FDA does and what the public thinks it does are as different as night and day."

Since much research is paid for by the industry, one can imagine that it takes immense courage to contradict the sweetener manufacturers and their advocates. The sweetener market is global and unfair to consumers because it is based on laws that are out of proportion. There is no good reason to voluntarily ingest aspartame. This food product creates a sickly need for starchy foods and makes you fat. This is what Dr. Roberts clearly explained to his patients, specifying that aspartame is particularly dangerous for diabetics. When they stopped consuming aspartame, their average weight loss was 10 kilos per person. However, the American and European legislations, which are supposed to protect health, maintain that aspartame is suitable for dieting and they always assure its non-toxicity.

4 - Legislation, lobbies and blocking

The American FDA legislation is based on the old Searle cheat sheet. EFSA, the European regulatory body, is sovereign and also states that aspartame is safe. The reason why pure aspartame is no longer sold is that it has been replaced by sucralose or stevia extract. More powerful sweeteners such as advantame, also approved by the EFSA, are not well known. Its sweetness is thirty thousand times higher than that of sugar. Consumers can only note the apathy of public authorities to really want to verify their safety. Whether aspartame or its more potent replicas are perceived as harmless or fatal does not matter to the manufacturers. Their lobby defends them with reassuring, often fallacious and sometimes grotesque arguments. "Wisdom does not enter into a malicious soul and science without conscience is only the ruin of the soul", said Rabelais, humanist physician. The profiteers of credulity do not have to fear our laws because no *class action* is on the horizon, the only weapon capable of forcing the industry to a bit of ethics. The art of the lobbies is to create the hope of a better physical form, then to block the road to any "useless" question.

Many official experts, directly paid by the industry, support an old lie, without batting an eyelid. E951 and its cousin E969 allow for a light sweet tooth, that's all we should remember. And when the press tries to deconstruct the mystification in a cyclical way, it is unable to explain the insidious ravages due to aspartame because the evaluations at charge have not been retained... But in a world of zapping where many advertisers use the incriminated sweeteners in their products, can we really go deeper into the subject ?

For the past thirty years, aspartame has been killing people all over the world, but no one is really worried about it. There has been no worldwide epidemiological study, so brain tumors, Alzheimer's disease and other ailments are not counted as attributable to the chemistry of sweeteners once ingested. Some diseases are particularly progressing where diet food is established, but the French Federation of Diabetics (FFD) is pleased "that the controversies on aspartame are finally lifted", which had sown doubt and mistrust among consumers. Since EFSA concluded that aspartame is safe, the risks, such as carcinogenesis, mutagenesis, alteration of the central nervous system, disorders of cognitive functions in adults and children, abnormalities of fetal development, would be completely removed. EFSA claims to have taken into account all available information. However, there is no authority to verify its good faith, because it is the supreme authority that grants or not its "blessing" to a product. As for the major soda brands, they continue to adorn aspartame with its benefits, synonymous with health and body care. The October 2012 study by the International Sweeteners Association (ISA) was also conducted on behalf of the French Federation of Diabetics. It is this kind of conflict of interest that is unacceptable if one considers that one cannot be both judge and jury. The Sweeteners organization applauded after the "verdict" of the EFSA in favor of an unchanged Daily Intake of aspartame, by publishing this text:

"Brussels, 10 December 2013. - EFSA, in a scientific opinion made public today and following a re-evaluation process of aspartame, started in 2011, confirms once again the safety of aspartame for all, children, adults, pregnant women... ISA welcomes a decision that corroborates the conclusions of more than 600 scientific works over forty years, in accordance with the scientific consensus on this sweetener.

Aspartame is a safe ingredient

EFSA experts have conducted a thorough evaluation of all available scientific data on aspartame and concluded today that the consumption of aspartame is safe for everyone.

EFSA states in its press release, "The experts of the ANS panel took into account all available information and, after a thorough analysis, concluded that the acceptable daily intake of 40 mg/kg body weight/day is adequately protective for the general population." The opinion makes clear that the breakdown products of aspartame (phenylalanine, methanol, and aspartic acid) are also naturally present in other foods (methanol, for example, is found in fruits and vegetables).

"In this debate more ideological than scientific, the unqualified conclusions issued today by EFSA on aspartame will reassure the French who were wondering about the subject," said Dr. Hervé Nordmann, chairman of the Scientific Committee of ISA France.

"Consumer health has always been a priority for ISA's industry members," he adds."

Every word counts. And the investigation should end there. But let's take up the language: decomposition methanol is indeed found in fruit, but who is going to eat the skin of a rotten banana? Let's remember that methanol is the poison that once caused blindness or death in some alcoholics. It is considered a cumulative poison because of its low degree of elimination. It oxidizes into formaldehyde and formic acid. The famous doctor Nordmann mentioned above must know this, even though he is paid by the manufacturers of aspartame. At the time of his statement, he was working for Industry Council for Development (ICD) and Ajinomoto. In a dossier "Aspartame, controversial studies", he declared that "aspartame could solve many health problems", signing Dr Hervé Nordmann, head of the aspartame committee of the International Sweeteners Association. He was at the heart of advertising inserts and in the organization chart of certain lobbies. Present at ICD, he represented the industry and not veterinary or human medicine. ICD is linked to the FAO, the United Nations Food and Agriculture Organization. ICD presents itself as a private, non-profit company, but its representatives all belong to the sweetener industry. Their spokesperson, Dr. Nordmann wrote *Avec ou sans*, a book published in 2014 by Cherche midi, whose banner is "Finally the truth about aspartame". For the author, these are "trials in infamy" that are made to this brave aspartame by the sugar lobbies, the media and social networks.

At this stage of the investigation, it is good to recall Article 13 of the Code of Medical Ethics: "When a doctor participates in an action of public information, he must report only confirmed data, exercise caution and be concerned about the repercussions of his words to the public."

The same is true for the ethics that journalists must respect. The Charter of Professional Ethics for Journalists states that "The public's right to quality, complete, free, independent and pluralist information, recalled in the Declaration of Human Rights and the French Constitution, guides journalists in the exercise of their mission. This responsibility towards the citizen takes precedence over any other."

However, the specialized press[16] often chooses reassuring headlines about aspartame and it is difficult for ordinary people to face a well-oiled rhetoric. Toxicologist Gérard Pascal, an expert in food culture and who had responsibilities in teaching and research at INRA, is wary of "disinformation", but of that of "non-experts": "Why panic the population?" he declared to Ouest-France in 2011, speaking of aspartame. Is it a coincidence that he received the Ajinomoto Association's Nutrition Research Award in 2006? One thing is certain, he was president of the scientific council of the French Agency for Food Safety (AFSSA) from 1999 to 2002 and he was chairing the scientific council when the agency was asked to reassess the risks of aspartame, after the publication of a study establishing links between consumption and brain cancer. In an official report dated May 7, 2002, the AFSSA cleared aspartame. Finally, why worry and panic the population, since the "experts" tell us that they are watching over our health. We must then ask ourselves: what if the fake sugar lobby was sincere? What if additives and sweeteners were not dangerous? One could then think that the lobbies are perfectly playing their role as purveyors of healthy products through impartial, scrupulous and educational scientists. For the moment, the diet lobby can push to consumption without

---

16. Examples: *Le Quotidien du médecin*: "L'aspartame n'est pas dangereux, confirme l'Agence européenne"; website Doctissimo: "Aspartame: après réévaluation, l'EFSA conclut à l'absence de risque".

fear of being pinned down. But would we voluntarily eat a product that, once ingested, would become formic acid and would attack our grey matter? In order to sort out the true from the false, we have to tackle highly technical cross-sections; but before the scientific truth sheds light on our choices, torrents of *sweet light* will have taken their toll on some of us. In reality, cowardice and collusion always hide the substance of the matter. The FDA was the first to be manipulated. FDA investigator Arthur M. Evangelista[17] expressed concern that aspartame caused impaired brain function, nerve damage, and systemic organ complications, but that greed prevailed. According to him, it was not a question of responsible science, but of profit and power:

"As an American who trusts the system we all created, as an American who used to work for it, it made me angry! Public health has taken a backseat to greed. Greed is the "engine" that perpetuates this epidemic: the collusion of our government with the influence of a multinational conglomerate. Dr. G. D. Searle approached Dr. Harry Waisman, biochemist, professor of pediatrics, director of the University of Wisconsin, Joseph P. Kennedy Jr. an expert known for his knowledge of phenylalanine toxicity and mental retardation, to conduct a study on the effects of aspartame on primates. The study was initiated on January 15, 1970 and was completed on or about April 25, 1971. Dr. Waisman died unexpectedly in March 1971... The actual results were concealed from the FDA...G. D. Searle denied any knowledge of the involvement or initiation, design, or execution of the study...A number of false statements were made by G. D. Searle..."

The first falsification was American and it contaminated the world. The scientist Betty Martini wrote an open letter to Mr. Jeffrey Moon, of the European Food Safety Authority, following the EFSA opinion. She accuses the sweetener industry of illicit agreement with EFSA! Her letter summarizes the questions about

---

17. James Bowen and Arthur M. Evangelista, "Brain Cell Damage from amino acid isolates: A primary concern from aspartam-based products and artificial sweetening agents," May 6, 2002, read at http://www.qualityassurance.synthasite.com

4 - Legislation, lobbies and blocking

the locks that prevent a real transparency[18]. The calls for caution are worldwide, but the lobbies do not care about investigations that are not favorable to them. We can see ILSI[19] in action in Europe protecting its products. This organization was created by members belonging to the chemical, food and pharmaceutical industries. However, ILSI is directly linked to EFSA whose role is to judge the harmfulness or harmlessness of consumer products. The International Life Sciences Institute is an essential piece of the puzzle. This institute started in 1978 by studying caffeine as a food additive. Its academic members work on specific topics: functional foods and obesity. The ISLI, which has a worldwide presence, studies, among other things: the merits and acceptable doses for additives and pesticides in Europe; sweetness and satiety, comparison with or without low-calorie sweeteners; sweeteners in children to fight obesity; sweeteners for adult diets; "sweetness" receptors and brain circuits; caries prevention; risks of using plants in food (Natural Toxin Task Force of ILSI Europe), etc.

When aspartame was introduced, the diet marketers kept talking about its almost magical ability to make people lose weight. To encourage women to smoke, didn't the tobacco companies tell them that Slim, a brand of cigarettes dedicated to women, would make them slimmer? Not false, but the tobacco also causes the cancer of the lungs... And so much the worse if today the aspartame ruins with low noise the health insurance.

---

18. See Appendix 2.

19. The International Life Sciences Institute (ILSI) was created in 1978 at the initiative of large American food companies such as Heinz, Procter & Gamble, General Foods and Kraft Foods. This lobby group was initially largely controlled by Coca-Cola. From 1991 onwards, ILSI was headed by Alex Malaspina, one of the vice presidents of the Atlanta-based multinational. ILSI's funding sources then diversified among the main multinationals in the food industry (Coca-Cola, Danone, Kraft Foods, Ajinomoto (world leader in food additives), the chemical industry (BASF, Dow Chemicals, DuPont...), pesticides and GMOs (Monsanto, Bayer CropScience, Syngenta...), detergents (Procter & Gamble, Unilever), drugs (Pfizer, Merck...), and even oil (Exxon Mobil). (Source: ILSI Annual Report 2011). With the exception of Antarctica, all continents are home to an ILSI branch, with headquarters in Washington. This includes manufacturers or users of aspartame. ILSI members also belong to the biotechnology and related industries, including cosmetics. Its European office opened in Brussels in 1986.

When Monsanto acquired G. D. Searle, it separated Searle Pharmaceuticals and NutraSweet Company and abandoned the simple coli that produced aspartame for boosted *Escherichia coli*: larger, more productive GMO E. coli. The powder from the drying of these genetically modified bovine fecal bacteria is called the "silent killer" by its critics. Does it cause the *Classic Methanol Neural Tube Defect*? That's not the question yet. The law allows the sale of aspartame and the manufacturers green their image so that they are not suspected of anything. Thus AminoSweet sings its own "merits". By producing aspartame instead of sugar, this company defends nature, arguing that the manufacture of sweeteners avoids the waste of millions of cubic meters of water, unlike the manufacture of cane sugar for example: real *green washing* supporting marketing. As for health, it is hardly noticeable when it is "wasted"... When insurance companies will tackle the subject, we will see more clearly. In the meantime, the lobbies are offering grants to improve their image, are fictitious the studies of many researchers and are constantly polishing their image in the medical community.

ILSI says it, the followers say it: you can take in a kilo of aspartame a year and drink dozens of diet cans a day... Scientists say that a man weighing 80 kilos can ingest 400 mg of saccharin, 560 mg of cyclamate, 1,200 mg of acesulfame-K and 3,200 mg of aspartame every day without any risk to his health. We'd like to see them in action... The aspartame lobbyists have not only sales people giving lectures, but toxicologists as well. Ms. Bernadene Magnuson is an example of "perfect" industry casting. And here's how Coca-Cola puts it: "Millions of people around the world regularly consume food and beverages with aspartame that they love, some for more than 30 years. Some are asking for more information. Does it increase appetite, for example? To clarify scientifically, the Coca-Cola Beverage Institute For Health & Wellness asked toxicology expert Dr. Bernadene Magnuson to share with health care professionals what they need to know when asked questions by aspartame consumers."

Between 2008 and 2009, Magnuson, an academic specializing in nanotechnology in animal feed, gave numerous lectures. At a seminar in Auckland on "Aspartame, Fact and Fiction"[20], when asked the awkward question of whether aspartame is safe for pregnant women, she replied, "It's not dangerous for pregnant or nursing women or for children. In addition, it is very good for fighting obesity." Asked specifically how much of it is left in the bloodstream, she replied, "There is much more danger in eating a banana containing methanol." The banana is definitely a good thing! According to Dr. Bernadene Magnuson, aspartame drinks leave less aspartic acid, phenylalanine and methanol in the bloodstream than a banana, a tomato, or a *smoothie*. This consultant's interview is worth listening to in its entirety. Despite rare hearings seriously organized to hear anti-aspartame, the industry defends itself through this kind of consultant. Nobody replies to her, even if it is about aspartic acid, which is involved in gluconeogenesis, but which is known to be an excitatory neurotransmitter in the brain, activating the glutamate receptors. D-aspartic acid, as well as its salt, sodium D-aspartate, have moreover anabolic properties... But, oh astonishment, EFSA used arguments of Dr Magnuson, Coca-Cola's lawyer, also member of the Burdock group[21] and of a group of experts, financed by Ajinomoto in 2007... What needed to be demonstrated is: some experts are openly paid by the manufacturers This is called pantouflage or intellectual laziness. As for the Burdock group to which Mrs Magnuson belongs, it publishes a host of reports that EFSA in turn uses. In the field of carcinogenesis, for example, the choice was made of a negative partial study from 1981 by Hiroji Ishii, carried out by the Ajinomoto laboratory, on brain cancer, which refutes three studies carried out by the Italian Ramazzini Institute, which Dr. Magnuson

---

20. "Aspartame, facts and fiction'seminars held in Auckland and Wellington, featuring Canadian toxicologist, Dr. Bernadene Magnuson and Foundation Secretary, nutritionist, Nikki Hart. In partnership with Coca-Cola and Network Communications. Nikki Hart promotes *Diet Coke as a* nutritionist. Video interview with Dr. Magnuson on aspartame.net. Dr. Magnuson is now part of the Global Stevia Institute (GSI) and on the Coca-Cola 2017 website, she answers all your questions.

21. This group prepares the files that the FDA must target, for example the attribution of GRAS (*Generally Recognized As Safe*). Read Adrian Chang's testimony that 56 of the 90 studies opposing aspartame were not cited by Ajinomoto in the report to the Burdock panel. For Magnuson's response, read her article, "Carcinogenicity of Aspartame in Rats Not Proven," on the Environmental Health Perspectives website.

is also attacking. EFSA preferred to consult the Burdock group, a group of lawyers and experts, rather than independent institutes. So the *believers* can sleep easy... What the consumer wants is to be able to compare different opinions by himself, but he knows little or nothing about the subject. In the past, for example, 900 kilos of sugar were needed as a preservative for one ton of antibiotics, today only 15 kilos of aspartame are needed. It is so profitable that 100% of industrial studies are in favor of aspartame, whether or not it is mixed with other substances. This market therefore decides alone and turns its back on the contradictory results that expose the effects of aspartame: in particular the cerebral malformations of infants, autism, metabolic disorders and neurological effects at doses corresponding to those to which the human population is exposed.

Aspartame in all its forms is flooding the markets worldwide. It is sold, recommended "for a better life", a "clinical nutrition without problems". Consumers are encouraged to believe in an industrial Santa Claus and a protective mother medicine. At little cost, they are made to swallow all the sweeteners in the world and then expensive drugs in case of problems, which sometimes also contain them... Many fibromyalgias, autoimmune and neurodegenerative diseases, are undoubtedly linked to the chemistry of sweeteners. Emerging diseases have multifactorial origins, but nobody dares to ask the question: what about aspartame in all this?

5 - Reasons for a persistent silence

"We only know a priori what we ourselves put into things. This phrase from Immanuel Kant illustrates that without studying the ramifications between industry, politics and public health, we cannot pin down aspartame.

Many of the well-known figures[22] in the United States have worked for Monsanto and the federal government. Some of them fought for the truth before turning their backs. If we take only Monsanto, this group knows how to muzzle through "donation", funding for example the American Diabetic Association, the American Dietetic Association and the American College of Physicians Conference... In 2016, its contribution to electoral campaigns was close to 80% in favor of the Republicans and exceeded 20% for the Democrats. Its generous pincers extend to the world. Patronage and permissive laws bound the perimeter of access to the real subject. The aspartame business benefits so many industries that scientists with integrity seem to be preaching in the wilderness. What seems crazy is that the FDA still finds no downside to baking aspartame and even approved aspartame in baby milk in early 2013, without any mandatory mention! Yet, phenylalanine can cause mental retardation in babies with phenylketonuria. A petition addressed to the FDA was concerned about this...

---

22. David Beier, William Conlon, Sam Skinner, Robert Fraley, Michael A. Friedman, Marcia Hale, Arthur Hull Hayes, Jonh L. Henshaw, Rob Horsch, Michael Kantor, Gwendolyn S. King, Richard J. Mahoney, Margaret Miller, George Poste, William D. Ruckelhaus, Donald Rumsfeld, Suzanne Sechen, Robert B. Shapiro, Islam Siddiqui, Michael Taylor, Charles Thomas, Clerance Thomas, Anne Veneman, Jack Watson, Seth Waxman, Virginia Weldon, Rufus Yerxa, etc.

Two thirds of the American population ingest aspartame, including 40% of children. The overweight is not related to the average 3,700 calories/day, it is related to something else, because otherwise, the Italians and the French would be as obese as the Americans. This indicates that Europeans probably have a better lifestyle, that they walk more and have a more varied diet, but that advertisements everywhere are lying when they say that dieting helps to slim down or keep the figure without mentioning the long-term risks. The silence goes on and on, probably because aspartame is considered as a safe food additive and not as a medicine, and because doctors do not consider it as a drug, a poison, or even an allergenic product, but as an anti-calorie crutch... Yet aspartame makes people fat, diabetologists should say to themselves if they study the world obesity curves. Nearly 100 million Chinese have become obese because they have changed their way of eating... The percentage of obese people in the world follows more or less the consumption of diet. If some doctors call it a "food Mediator", lobbies are acting in Brussels, in the parliaments of the European Union member countries, to put out the fire of questions. They have nothing to fear from the food safety agencies. The European Food Safety Agency (EFSA), based in Parma, advises the EFSA and is based on industry scientific literature. Several members of its board, scientific council and expert panels for food additives are accused of having conflicts of interest with industry because of their relationship with ILSI. The EFSA, which should inform EFSA, has dismissed independent scientific productions on the basis of controversial criteria[23]. Without a totally independent international authority, millions of young people will become obese and *sweet light* will have reinforced their appetite for sweeteners. A little explanation: if the pancreas after too much sugar ingested provides satiety, sweeteners do not provoke any disgust after a diet of light. Advertising has even insidiously introduced itself into our French school books. (139 brands

---

23. In December 2011, anticipating a damning prejudgment report by the European Court of Auditors on its practices, and put under pressure by the European Parliament, the EASA would have redefined its independence policy, particularly with regard to the scientific basis of its decisions and conflicts of interest whether scientific, political, economic or religious.

including 7 beverages). Danone, Kellogs, Nestlé even advertise in some primary school classes[24]. Without any embarrassment, brands offer their drinks even in universities, and this is called partnership. However, American researchers claim that frogs ingesting aspartame become confused and suffer from methanol poisoning. On the other hand, phenylalanine derived from aspartame decreases serotonin and can cause bipolar episodes and tendencies to suicide and depression, they say, but there are few studies about "aspartame-addicted" youth. Protective authorities create a blur that allows silence.

In 2009, EFSA reaffirmed that "there was no reason to revise the acceptable daily intake previously established for aspartame", keeping silent on the brain risks. But in 2011, she told the European Parliament that she had never had the famous studies in front of her! The industry that provided them did not have the industrial studies in its possession either. EFSA wrote however: "Following thorough safety assessments, aspartame has been considered safe for human consumption. This is called drowning the fish or sweeping the dust under the carpet! The few opponents did not make the weight. Why not?

EFSA is governed by a Management Board that must be appointed jointly by the EU Member States and the European Parliament. In reality, members are "chosen" from a shortlist of candidates, following a public call for expressions of interest. Four of the 14 members of the Management Board must "have experience in organizations representing consumer and other interests in the food chain", which is not the case since, according to EFSA itself, two of these four experts come from the industry[25].

Diana Banati, who was a member of the ILSI board, resigned after the controversy over her links with industry. Milan Kovas, a member of the EFSA board was a member of ILSI, Jiri Ruprich, of the Danone Institute...

---

24. See the work of Paul Ariès, political scientist, University of Lyon II.

25. At the time of this investigation, these were Matthias Horst, director of the German Food and Beverage Federation, and Piet Vanthemsche, who heads the Flemish Industrial Farmers' Union and holds a management position in the Agri Investment Fund, with shares in 19 agribusiness-related companies.

And who, for the preliminary toxicological tests? An EFSA toxicologist, also a consultant for the food industry, member of ILSI. The loop is closed from the inside, in all opacity. Experts easily infiltrate and offer the services of the industry until this entrism becomes too obvious. The chairwoman and vice-chairwoman of the expert group, Mrs. Ivonne Rietjens, has received money for her laboratory from Nestlé since 2005, and from the International Organization of Taste (IOFI) since 2010. She has also worked for BASF. She has been a member of the Flavour Extract Manufacturers Association of which Coca-Cola and Pepsi-Cola are very active members, and she has also worked with ILSI to redefine risk assessment procedures for food and chemicals. This goes beyond expertise, cronyism, it reflects collusion, which is defined as "a secret agreement between two or more persons to act in fraud of another's rights, and which is punishable by law."

But this law is not enforced. Ms. Rietjens' fellow Dutchman, group rapporteur Gerrit Speijers, has been a consultant for Danone and PepsiCo International since 2010, and has also worked with ILSI Europe.

The Austrian Jürgen Köning was a consultant for Danone. The Belgian Paul Tobback has been a member of the scientific committee of the Belgian industry lobby since 2001 and for the Carrefour chain. The Irishwoman Iona Pratt has worked with ILSI. British businessman John Gilbert and French scientist Jean-Charles Leblanc have both been advisors to ILSI or have worked for ILSI. Toxicology professor Dominique Parent-Massin worked as a consultant for Coca-Cola in 2009, as well as for Ajinomoto. In March 2011, she declared financial ties to Ajinomoto that were considered a conflict of interest by EFSA.

When some of the experts were renewed in 2011, two of the five new experts, Ricaro Crebelli and Ursula Gundert-Remy forgot to refer to their jobs as consultants for ILSI (the ILSI working group was headed by a Monsanto employee and included employees from Cargill, Bayer and Syngenta).

Chairman Harry Kuiper[26], has been active in ILSI for at least a decade. He has been chairman of the EFSA GMO Panel since 2003.

---

26. Kuiper has changed his EFSA declaration of interest to exclude his most recent ILSI connections.

Joe Perry, the group's former vice president for GMOs, was paid by a subcontractor of BASF, Bayer, Monsanto and Syngenta[27]. Until 2006, Perry was a researcher for a private institute sponsored by Syngenta, Bayer, DuPont and Dow AgroSciences.

Jeremy Sweet, with the predestined name, former vice president of the GMO group, received funding from Monsanto, Bayer and BASF in 2006. He has also done seminars in Japan and Korea for ILSI. Since 1995 he has been a member of the British Crop Protection Association, a lobby for the biotech industry. Joachim Schiemann[28], a member of the GMO group and the Public Research and Regulation Initiative - an industry lobby group that seeks to relax environmental protection legislation - was fired from EFSA.

Jean-Michel Wal received funding from Nestlé and was a member of an ILSI working group. He was also a member of the French Institute for Nutrition.

Detlef Bartsch was a consultant for Monsanto. He wrote an article with employees of Monsanto, Dupont, Syngenta, BASF with his colleagues of the GMO expert group.

Jozsef Kiss had his laboratory funded by Pioneer Hi-Bred to test the environmental impact of GMO corn.

Patrick du Jardin was a paid consultant to Monsanto in 2006.

Howard Davies is a GMO potato researcher, and his institute was funded by Monsanto to introduce GMO potatoes to Kenya. He has also had external contracts with BASF and Bayer, and has lectured for ILSI.

As for the EFSA working group on "The threshold of toxicological concern", 10 of its 13 members have conflicts of interest, according to the Pesticide Action Network. Strangely, it was set up at the initiative of its chair, Susan Barlow, a British consultant for the chemical industry, who had clients such as ILSI, Pfizer or PepsiCo. All expert groups are affected. The EFSA does not seem credible to talk to us about aspartame... It is a world that lives in almost permanent isolation and that brings together people often

---

27. Syngenta is also involved in the Gates Foundation›s Svalbard Global Seed Vaul project, a gene bank created in 1984.

28. Biography on https://www.testbiotech.org/sites/default/files/Testbiotech_Schlecht_Beraten_3.pdf

linked to one or more interdependent industrialists. Where can impartial research on the effects of E951 be found, and how can rare experts of integrity have authority, trapped in such a mesh created by lobbies? The joint report by Corporate Europe Observatory and Europe Open Source shows that "most industry studies used in the regulatory process are not peer-reviewed or published. They fall into the category of 'grey literature', documents whose reliability remains unknown."

It is clear that EFSA is more than connected to industry. Yet all regulatory institutions have virtually the same experts as the lobbies and do not care about the demands for transparency[29]. EFSA has vehemently denied the accusations it has been targeted with, in particular of being infiltrated. Its executive director, Catherine Geslain-Lanéelle, said the reports contained "factual errors" and "misled the public about EFSA. A weak defense, but Ms. Geslain-Lanéelle, appointed director general of agricultural, agri-food and territorial policies, soon had no more to explain[30]. In her official CV in the Hollande government, her time at EFSA was not mentioned. This body looks like a springboard or a private club, but not an exemplary organization. In a complaint about two new experts failing to declare links with ILSI, EFSA said, "In accordance with EFSA's policy on declarations of interest, the experts were not required to declare these activities as they are not related to the field of activity of their scientific panel." An article in Le *Monde* criticized EFSA and its intricacies through revelations by José Bové: "The chairwoman of the European Food Safety Authority's management board is also a member of the board of an association of the largest agribusiness companies. This is the revelation made by José Bové, Member of the European Parliament (Europe Ecology), at a press conference in Brussels on Wednesday, September 29, 2010. The documents

---

29. Kartika Liotard, the MEP responsible for liaising between EFSA and the Parliament, has repeatedly called for new research or the use of other research for years, without result.

30. The executive director explained this and yet declared in an article in Le *Monde* in January 2012, "I say it strongly, EFSA is not infiltrated by industry." The European Food Safety Authority had been accused of a lack of transparency and links between experts and industry. Until now, Catherine Geslain-Lanéelle was director general of the DGPE, and in 2017 she was appointed director of the cabinet of Jacques Mézard, Minister of Territorial Cohesion.

presented show that Diana Banati, the president of the board of directors, concealed the fact that she also belonged to the board of directors of ILSI Europe (International Life Sciences Institute), a body in which she rubs shoulders with representatives of ten major companies such as Kraft Foods, Nestlé or Danone.

In a press release of the same day, José Bové called for the resignation of Ms. Diana Banati, who has since left EFSA due to conflicts of interest, and who had no problem finding another position. At the heart of this entanglement between industries and EFSA, Prof. Erik Millstone of the Freeman Center in Sussex, spoke in late December 2013 of inconsistency regarding the panels chosen by EFSA in its re-evaluation of aspartame as a food additive. He questioned the credibility of scientific arguments, while most of the negative opinions were not taken into account. He reported on 15 studies, three of which were alarming regarding the mortality rate of laboratory rats. Sheets concerning the blindness of guinea pigs were not included. Professor Millstone sent the Bressler report and his own investigation. A document from the *Wall Street Journal,* which can be consulted on the Internet[31], puts the interests at stake into perspective. There was indeed a criminal investigation against NutraSweet, and the Searle company had indeed falsified the results. So EFSA, FDA same fight? These organizations are joined by ILSI, which denies being a pressure group[32]. As for the IFN (French Institute for Nutrition), it is a lobby whose members include the National Association of Food Industries, the Center for Sugar Studies and Documentation, the National Federation of Fat Industries, and multinationals such as Coca-Cola France, Danone, Kraft Foods, Kellogg's France, Nestlé or Unilever. But don't worry about the medical side if dieting makes you gain

---

31. *Wall Street Journal,* Feb. 7, 1986: "It is learned that two former prosecutors investigating Searle have been interviewed as witnesses by Andy Pasztor and Joe Davidson in Washington: they are two government lawyers who are determined to attack the maker of NutraSweet, accused of falsifying test results during the criminal and senatorial investigations against it."

32. Its current members are: Bayer, Coca-Cola, Danone, Kellogg's, Kraft Foods, Monsanto, Pepsi, Unilever, BASF, Cargill, Ferrero, Nestlé, Red Bull, Procter & Gamble, L'Oréal, Bio Mérieux, Brystol Myers Squibb, Exxon Mobil, Eli Lilly, Merck & Co, Novartis, Sanofi Aventis... On the board of directors, we find the president of Coca-Cola Europe, doctors from Kraft Foods, Sanofi Aventis, Monsanto, Syngenta, Danone, Nestlé, and some academics.

weight, diabetic diets are better supported with sweeteners, explains Dr. Pierre Azam: "The more tools we have to improve the quality of life, the easier it is to get our messages of respect for the rules of hygiene and diet across. His study, "Diabetics and Sweeteners," written for AFD and ISA USA (International Sweetener Association) was conducted from October 12 to 21, 2012, among 506 representative diabetics (types 1 and 2[33]) aged 15 years and older. Nutritionist Pierre Azam founded an association to fight obesity: the Obesity Observatory (OBOBS) and he claims that aspartame is a therapeutic weapon[34] to manage diabetes. And how does it fight obesity? Through the International Sweetener Association. It is through such doctors that aspartame is considered appropriate, so one is led to wonder why even diabetologists are unaware of the purpose of this investigation: diet is fattening! Patients are being cheated by their disease specialists, and the expert battles become a boon for the sweetener market, as they drag on. As obesity gains ground exponentially, the drug industry will follow... Health protection authorities should be exemplary and not cover up such aberrations. The last director chosen for the FDA by President Obama was Dr. Margaret Ann Hamburg, from Chicago, who declared that she wanted to finally ban the *shadow industry*, but it seems that she did nothing to ban aspartame. Dr. Roberts had also written to her, stating that he had long been concerned about "the negative and powerful effects of the chemical aspartame found in many 'sugar-free' products and consumed by half the population. This therapist with no ties to any company was clear: "The magnitude of this problem is startling. My own data includes the study of 1,400 people who have suffered serious disorders that can be directly attributed to the use of these products. Almost all of the cases are detailed in the 1,000 pages of my book *Aspartame Disease: An Ignored Epidemic*. A brochure accompanies this ignored epidemic, and other books are listed on my publisher's website Sunshine Sentinel Press Inc. Revelations of other aspartame-induced complications are being uncovered every week."

---

33. Type 1 diabetes is inherent to the person who suffers from an often hereditary diabetes, type 2 diabetes is related to a poor diet, a lack of physical activity.
34. 2012: *Top santé, Journal des Femmes*. 2013: *Destination Santé*.

Dr. Roberts was not heard. The Don Quixotes of health care are no match for the old cronies[35] that start in college and grow into powerful government networks. When lobbies easily approach FDA experts or people close to the White House, the industry can impose silence around a product. In France, lobbyists contact our deputies and senators, and the industry tries to get some press to show its credentials and convince them of the benefits of E951.

In *Marketing Magazine* n° 34 of November 1, 1998, the journalist Valérie Mitteaux had collected the words of the director of Monsanto's "mass consumption" department. He declared at the time:

"Our future lies in the field of nutrition. With products designed to improve people's well-being or to prevent diseases. Our objective is to develop products that will help compensate for, and prevent, the onset of these diseases linked to genetic inheritance. Today, we are able to develop products that fight against cholesterol."

The reporter then asked the question, "Are you going to innovate in the area of sweeteners?"

"Yes, they will change their packaging. But the major innovations will come from new sweeteners, successors to aspartame. In particular, our group has discovered a new molecule: neotame. It is due to be launched in the United States in the first quarter of 1999. This sweetener has a much higher sweetening power than aspartame. It has the particularity to resist to cooking. But also to be a taste enhancer: the taste of the product that you sweeten - tea, coffee... - comes out very superior to that of a coffee or tea sweetened with aspartame. That's pretty impressive. For the first time, Diet Coke has a real Coke taste. In a way, we find the natural origin of the taste.

The journalist then asked if aspartame had been definitively demonized. The answer was: "The negative rumors persist. Creativity on the subject is important! To counter this, we built a communication program aimed at specialized journalists and the medical profession, explaining the particularity of the molecule and the fact that it is perfectly digested by the body. This scientific communication program has enabled us to convince prescribers of the safety

---

35. One such network of wealthy students remains Skulls and Bones where former students now navigate politics and industry.

and benefits of the product. We are maintaining it with respect to the medical profession because there are always new sources of rumor."

For this Monsanto representative, it was clear: "There is no food product in the world that has been more tested. More than 2,000 studies have been conducted on animals, men, women and children. They have always been very positive. Aspartame does not pose any problem. These are two amino acids that are already natural constituents of our diet. At the end of a normal meal, you have consumed 200 g of them. One tablet of Canderel is 20 mg more digested by your body. There is no trace. And that's what's made it so successful around the world compared to saccharin or other sweeteners."

Arnaud Steiger was proud of his company, which he considers to be "the Microsoft of biotechnologies" and of its new product, neotame. This artificial sweetener E961[36] was developed by Monsanto in collaboration with American universities. It should prevent the production of phenylalanine, which makes it possible to ingest it in people suffering from phenylketonuria. This suggests that aspartame sold as a panacea was already not that healthy, and that its long-term safety in humans is uncertain. Neotame leads us to the philosophy surrounding the manufacture of aspartame. In 2013, Monsanto had it manufactured at Senomyx. Senomyx is one of the Russian dolls of history that pushes its research in conjunction with Ajinomoto. This company bills itself as a pioneer in flavor boosters. PepsiCo also has ties to this biotech company that has been testing food additives including some embryonic kidney cells: HEK293 (for *Human Embryonic Kidney cells)* usually used in vaccines but would be found in some of their drinks. The

---

36. Approved in the United States in 2002, it was not marketed in Canada until 2007. José Manuel Barroso signed its marketing approval for Europe at the end of 2009. According to *Medical Revue* of September 2002, the approval of neotame is based on the results of 113 unpublished studies, in animals and in humans, submitted to the FDA. One study showed that the offspring of rats fed 1000 mg/kg/day showed reduced motor activity and ability to swim in a maze; but at 100 and 300 mg/kg/day, it was normal. Two rodent studies showed a decrease in total body weight gain that did not appear to be related to food consumption. In humans, doses of neotame up to approximately 90-100 mg/kg/day for 13 weeks were not associated with any clinical abnormalities.

only counterbalance to food chemistry remains the vigilance of consumers. "In the past, in France, attempts were made to tax palm oil and aspartame. Regarding aspartame, a special tax had been set by the senators at 30 euros per kilo for 2013. And who was it that arrived on his high horse to contest it? The Minister of Budget at the time, Jérôme Cahuzac[37], previously linked to pharmaceutical laboratories such as Fabre and Lilly (the latter being himself linked to Monsanto), opposed the two taxes, judging "that they should rather be included in the draft budget of the Social Security".

Aspartame leads to everything, as long as you don't get out of it. Take the example of Japan's Ajinomoto "taste of the future". This more than 100 year old industry worked with Kellogg's Co and Knorr, joined forces with General Foods, Gervais Danone, and then created Ajinomoto Eurolysine SAS in the United States (specialist in amino acids and cost reduction for animal feed). It should be noted again that aspartame is part of this market. The Japanese group establishes its cooperation with NutraSweet in Switzerland, created Ajinomoto sweeteners Europe, Ajinex in Indonesia, and in Russia, with the blessing of Vladimir Putin, Ajinomoto Genetika. Ajinomoto Genetika's researchers were looking for the best way to feed old knowledge: E. Coli micro-organisms before fermentation. At Genetika, they do use *Escherichia coli*[38], a Searle specialty enhanced by Monsanto with GMO bleeding bacilli. In 2010, Ajinomoto Genetika Research Institute (AGRI) saw its sales rise to $14.2 billion. What unsuspected connections, political and scientific, around aspartame so microscopic at first glance. Everywhere and nowhere, its multiple masks make it a product difficult to attack. The industrialists involved in sweeteners conceal information, then maintain their image of misunderstood respectability. For example, Monsanto donated funds to the Hudson Institute's Center for Global Food Issues, and what does its director say about sweeteners? Dennis T. Avery mocks "activists who blame aspartame and other non-caloric sweeteners for obesity. He calls them "non-deniers" who

---

37. In comparison, we owe Dominique Strauss-Kahn a veto for the purchase of Orangina by Coca-Cola (November 1999). Orangina now belongs to a Japanese group.
38. Bacterial strain of *Escherichia coli* VNII genetika 472T23.

don't want a cheap product in their Coke. He adds that "they attack aspartame as dangerous and that good people believe them". This research institute demonstrates that there is an "in-between" where people end up believing their own lies. In conclusion, personal implications, independent laboratories and honest politicians do not lead to a global change of course. An independent authority is needed to shed light on the fake sugar industry. Its silence is only the result of an old cowardice added to the strength of the seducing lobbies of vulnerable "specialists"... How many experts have succumbed? As for consumers, they prefer to trust, and we can understand them, but in the United States, some are rebelling and removing the "*t*" from *Diet, which* gives *Die*[39] , to express their displeasure on social networks. In order to stop the controversy, it would be utopian to demand a comparative and global epidemiological investigation. As long as international trade dictates its laws on our plates and in our medicine cabinets, it will be difficult to turn back. More than 100 countries have approved the food use of aspartame and only Venezuela refuses to sell Diet Coke. But "aspartamiser" being legal, many unaccounted diseases can thus intoxicate in silence. The verb "to aspartame" is not in the dictionary, but everyone will understand its meaning.

---

39. *Diet*: "diet" and *die*: "die".

SWEETENERS AND CONSUMERS

1 - Sweeteners in Foods and Medicines

One billion human beings, adults, elderly, children, babies, and many fetuses, ingest sweeteners. There are so many "E's" that it's confusing! The sweeteners written **in bold** are those to be wary of for medical reasons which will be explained in the section *below* entitled "HEALTH".

By doing your shopping, by studying the contents of your cupboards, medicine box and refrigerator, you will quickly realize the number of sweetened products, aspartamized, that you consume most often without your knowledge.

The numbering of the "E" will allow you to enter the "wonderful" world of food chemistry. Sweeteners are like mushrooms: some are edible, others are edible in small doses, and the last ones can be deadly for some people. Indeed, some pathologies formally forbid E951.

E950 acesulfame-K: potassium salt often associated with other sweeteners.

E951 aspartame: artificial sweetener created from *Escherichia coli*: complaints filed for adverse effects in the United States against Searle, then Monsanto. Now Ajinomoto is the main manufacturer. FDA and EFSA attest to its safety. Other studies highlight risks for pregnant women, fetuses, children, diabetics and consider it as a promoter of neurodegenerative diseases.

E952: cyclamic acid and cyclamates, calcium cyclamate, potassium cyclamate, sodium cyclamate. **Artificial sweeteners prohibited in the United States and the United Kingdom.**

E953 : isomalt, polyol derived from sucrose (fructose and glucose molecules).

E954 : saccharin and its salts : sodium, potassium and calcium saccharinates. Synthetic product via toluene. Considered as carcinogenic in the United States. Banned in France, Germany, Spain, Hungary, Portugal, Malaysia and Zimbabwe, and as a beverage additive in Israel, Peru, Taiwan and Fiji.

E955: sucralose, an intense artificial sweetener (Canderel, Splenda, Aqualoz brands) that is stable to heat unlike aspartame. The Scientific Committee on Food approved its use in 2000, but other studies highlight certain pathologies.

E956 : table sweetener, derived from aspartic acid, considered in the United States as without toxicological risk. Alitame (Pfizer).

E957 : thaumatin, intense and natural sweetener from the Ketemfe fruit : possible allergies

E958 : glycyrrhisic acid.

E959 : neohesperidin dihydrochalone NHDC.

E960 : steviol glycosides.

E961 : neotame : contains aspartic acid and phenylalanine.

E962: salt of asparatame-acesulfame: artificial sweetener made from aspartame and acesulfame K admitted since 2000 as being without risk but must include the following mention: "contains a source of phenylalanine" as for aspartame.

E963: tagatose: natural sweetener derived from milk with no harmful effect. No ADI because no risk.

E964 : polyglycitol syrup (polyol).

E965: maltitol and maltitol syrup (polyol or sugar alcohol that replaces sugar close to sugar).

E966 : lactitol (laxative polyol).

E967 : xylitol (birch extract).

E968: erythritol: natural sweetener that does not cause cavities).

E969: advantame. Controversial in the US (produced by Ajinomoto). EFSA has given its approval for marketing but "considers that a maximum limit of palladium and platinum should be included in the product specifications". It contains phenylalanine.

The suosan related to beta 4 aspartic acid, aspartame and alitame, recognized as toxic, has not been assigned an "E".

E171 : titanium dioxide is a colorant in the form of nanoparticles and is not a sweetener.

E1201: medicines and cosmetics contain this vinyl polymer. It is used to make blood plasma.

Not all "E's" are the same. "E" stands for sweeteners, color additives, or preservatives. E's also include flavor enhancers, waxes and hydrocarbons, gums and gases. Each "E" plays a role. The E900 (dimethicone) is an antifoaming agent found in beverages, it is not dangerous unless it is in the presence of formaldehyde or formaldehyde found in the decomposition of aspartame. Just this E900 is surprising, we can find as residues: lead, arsenic, mercury, and this simple additive was authorized in 2012 by Europe. The following list is not exhaustive. It indicates products containing aspartame in alphabetical order. It is only a brief overview to which everyone can add new names or sometimes cross them out, as some manufacturers prefer to remove aspartame from their products. But let's take the first sugar-free product on the list: Activia 0% fruit yogurt, and discover its components. In addition to skim milk and fruit: fructo-oligosaccharides, thickeners, flavors, three sweeteners: E951 (aspartame), E950 (acesulfame-K), E955 (sucralose); concentrated grape juice and two colorings: E120 (carmine), E160 c (paprika extract). But what does the advertising say: "Discover Activia 0%, all the smoothness of Activia and the flavor of its beautiful pieces of fruit with now 0% fat and 0% added sugars."

Of course, there is no added sugar, but sucralose is an organochlorine compound. At high doses on laboratory rats, we can see "just" an enlargement of the liver and kidneys, an impairment of the immune system, a shrinking of the spleen and the thymus, and finally a renal mineralization. This E955 can give rise to carcinogenic compounds when exposed to heat and is not completely evacuated by the body, but it is authorized since 2005 in Europe. We can add E951 to it, from which the aspartame lobby would like to remove the mention attached to it: "contains a source of phenylalanine". The International Sweeteners Association (ISA) continues its campaign with the European Union ... But all products containing aspartame must at least include the warning. This prevention is mandatory for foodstuffs.

Food products containing aspartame
- Activia 0
- Actimel
- Airwaves
- Beautifix Oenobiol
- Beers (Kriek)
- Sweets
- Canada dry
- Canderel and Culinaire Canderel
- Carrefour Stylesse fruit cocktail
- Light Chambourcy with fruit and fromage blanc
- Chicklets
- Cigarettes (almost all brands contain additives)[40]
- Chocoline
- Clorets without sugar
- Cherryade
- Diet Coke, without caffeine
- Coca-Cola Zero and *Diet Coke*
- Ice creams (some)
- Gayelord Hausser Chocolate Cream - 350g
- Danacol
- Delight O
- Dentine
- *Diet Coke*
- Cora Harmony
- Toothpaste
- Table sweeteners
- Table Sweetener U, 5x100 tablets (+ Acesulfame-K)
- Sweeteners Zoetsof Carrefour 300 tablets (+ acesulfame-K)
- Fresubin high calorie cream[41]

40. Read "Deadly tobacco in all its forms, World No Tobacco Day 2006, WHO", to know the list of unexpected ingredients: chocolate, acetaldehyde, licorice, sweeteners, acrolein or ethylene aldehyde, formaldehyde. Aldehyde is a compound of the carbonyl family. The simplest aldehyde is formaldehyde or formalin.
41. Donated in nursing homes by Fresenius Kabi brand specialized in clinical and vital nutrition for diabetics.

- Eldorado light fruit cocktail with sweeteners
- Equal
- Fanta light
- Fisherman
- Flamby
- Freedent
- Frisk fresh breath
- Cakes
- Gerlinéa meal replacement
- Haribo Tagada
- Hollywood without sugar
- Hermesetas gold (granules)
- Instaslim
- Klondike (ice cream bars)
- Lipton Iced tea light
- Mentos Gum
- Minci drink powder
- Minute Maid
- Modifast Strawberry Muesli
- Nestea
- Nicorette
- Niquitin 2 mg without sugar
- Nutrition 400
- Oasis Zero
- Orangina Light
- Orbit without sugar
- Vichy menthol tablets
- Poulain Ligne Gourmande (withdrawn from sale since 2014 by
  Catbury)
- PowerFresh
- Diet Pepsi
- Pepsi Max
- Red Bull Sugarfree, Red Bull Zero
- Ricola (almost all)
- Schweppes: the aspartame of the light is replaced in 2013 by
  sucralose.
- 7 Up light

- Slimfast
- Sour Cola Roller
- Splenda
- Steocar
- Lollipops (Chupa Chyps without sugar)
- Stimorol
- Taillefine Danone
- Via Strawberry Light Syrup
- Vichy pastilles
- Weight Watchers Raspberry Sour Buttermilk 5 dl
- Wrigleys chewing gum Doublemint
- Yoplait (Panier fruits en quartiers 0%)
- Sveltesse (Nestlé)
Etc.

To which, it is often necessary to add other sweeteners.

Aspartame is not considered as a remedy but it is found as an additive in 500 medicines listed in the Vidal. It is used as a preservative. It can be harmful alone, and dangerous depending on the diseases treated.

Lists of the most common drugs containing aspartame
- **Abilify** (The risks listed speak for themselves: "precautions are necessary in cases of diabetes, epilepsy, heart disease (old or recent myocardial infarction, angina pectoris, heart failure, heart rhythm disorders...), abnormal blood pressure, risk of thrombosis, difficulty swallowing, history of addiction to gambling, dementia in an elderly person, phenylketonuria (orodispersible tablet: presence of aspartame.)
- Advil
- Adiva
- Alka-Seltzer
- Alipuro (mouthwash)
- Amoxicillin Almus 1 g
- Amoxicillin Biogaran 1 g, Amoxillin Zentiva Lab, Agram Gé.

- Amoxycil/clav[42]
- Rhone Aspirin
- Augmentin 500 mg, powdered oral suspension **for adults, children and infants**
- Brexine granulated sachets
- Berocca effervescent
- Bisolvon
- Brexin
- Buccalsone
- Calcium 600
- Calcium Sandoz
- Cacit Vitamin D3 500 mg/440 IU, chewable tablet
- CB 12 (mouthwash)
- Centrum dietary supplement, 20 effervescent tablets, 60 tablets Centrum Junior (Pfizer group)
- **Celance** (Lilly) (**antiparkinsonian, stopped marketing secables in 2011**)
- Celestene 2 mg
- Clamoxyl
- Clavucid syrup 250
- Clozapine tablets 13.52 mg aspartame
- Dafalgan codeine
- **Diacomit** (or Stiripentol: **anti-epileptic**)
- D. Vital calcium efferdose
- Donepezil Sandoz
- Drill without sugar
- Eludril
- Fervex Child and Fervex Pheniramine Adult, sugar-free
- Fixical Vitamin D3 500 mg/400 IU and Calcium Vitamin D3
- Flustimex
- Fluxetine Cristers 20 mg
- Gaviscon,

---

42. This medication has precautions: AMOXICIL/CLAV 1G/125MG ZYD SAC 8. The therapeutic indications are accompanied by warnings: "Store at a temperature not exceeding 30°C. This drug SHOULD NEVER BE USED in case of allergy to any of the components of the drug, and due to the presence of aspartame (E951), this drug is contraindicated in cases of phenylketonuria."

1 - Sweeteners in foods and medicines

- Gavisconell chewable, sugar free
- Heet
- Imovax Polio (formaldehyde, found in Axavim against hepatitis A).
- Josacin 1,000 mg
- Klean-Prep
- Laroscorbine 500 mg without sugar
- Lysomucil effervescent
- MagneVie B6 express (Sanofi-Aventis advises that this product should not be exposed to heat (no more than 25°) or light).
- Metamucil
- **Methyline** without sugar effervescent: contraindication, in case of phenylketonuria, because of the presence of aspartame.
- **Motilium** (prescribed for nausea in children), **withdrawn from sale since January 19, 2012**, but not the one without aspartame. Motilium in effervescent granules contains it. It would have recently caused 150 sudden deaths that would be linked to this drug.
- Muco-X 600
- Moviprep
- Mupax, **withdrawn from sale since August 17, 2011**
- Naturlax
- Nicogum mint, sugar free
- Nicopass eucalyptus and licorice mint
- Nicotine Pierre Favre
- Niquitin without sugar
- Novabritin (Augmentin)
- Nuardin
- Ordipha 500
- Orocal Vitamin D3
- Orochol (Mutachol), cholera vaccine
- Perdolan mono C tablets and Junior
- Pixidin tablets
- Prednisolone Mylan
- Questran
- Questran sachets
- Rhinathiol

- Riperdal M Tab at all doses (antipsychotic)
- Romilar
- Singulair
- Soparyx in bags
- Solupred
- Soparyx
- Stellavit without sugar
- Steocar calcium
- Structocal Vitamin D3
- Takadol 100 mg (not recommended for epileptics and depressives)
- Tagamet
- Transilane without sugar
- Tilcotil effervescent
- Tylenol
- Totephan in bags
- **Vimpat** 200 mg and syrup (according to the Vidal: indicated in combination in the treatment of partial seizures with or without secondary generalization in adults and adolescents (16-18 years) with epilepsy).
- Vitamins Adiva, Vitame C Upsa
- Vitascorbol sugar-free buffered
- Vogalib 5mg without sugar, 7,5mg lyophilisat
- Zantac
- Zofran or Zophren
- Zomigoro
- Zonegran or Zonisamide (anti-epileptic)
- **Zyprexa** Velotab Lilly[43]

The problem with aspartame is its perilous interaction with drugs such as Depakine or Depakote: anti-epileptic drugs that have sadly made the news. But how do you know what is good, and at what

---

43. The laboratory is more precise than the Vidal: "There is no experience in children. ZYPREXA powder for injectable solution should not be used in children or adolescents due to a lack of data regarding safety and efficacy. In Contraindications: Patients with a known risk of angle closure glaucoma. Further: exacerbation of diabetes... Also contains propylene glycol." *Full* legal *disclaimer ZYPREXA CP, IM and VELOTAB.*

dosage, for one person, and bad for another? Aspartame interacts with all antidepressants and drugs like Ritalin, which is given to hyperactive children. It is not the substance itself, but its transformation into metabolites[44] in the body that will generate risks, and the metabolites lead to chain reactions whose scope is unknown.

Is it the aspartame in a drink or a drug that exacerbates diabetes and attacks the brain or rather its metabolites? Why does the Vidal list aspartame as an "excipient of note"? As long as it is not metamorphosed, aspartame seems harmless. What is it composed of before it undergoes transformation at body heat? Aspartame is composed of amino acids, and the problem before metabolites appear is phenylalanine (50%), aspartic acid (40%) and methanol (10%).

Let's remember that an intense sweetener brings neither calories nor nutrients, but rather disadvantages. Dr. Oz called sweeteners *head-fake foods*, in other words, lures that are not only tasty but also cerebral. Regarding the sweeteners and additives in tobacco, Stanton Glantz, professor of medicine and researcher at the Center for Tobacco Control Research and Education, (University of San Francisco), explained the scientific manipulation of this kind of addition in cigarettes. With three experts, he verified the conclusions of the research program conducted by Philip Morris that was supposed to prove the safety of additives added to its tobacco. In the late 1990s, Philip Morris was concerned about the possibility of an intrusion in its data by the FDA. In anticipation of this, the tobacco company had launched *Project MIX*, which was supposed to evaluate the additional toxicity of 333 of the 599 additives added to tobacco in order to attest to the absence of overtoxicity of these adjuvants and other flavouring agents. The conclusion was: no new effects attributable to these additives. But according to the findings of Stanton Glantz and his team, if one looks at the total amount of toxics produced by inhaled combustion and not released, more than 20% of the toxics are formed by fifteen known carcinogens and cytotoxics. There have been no studies of the fate of high-temperature heated sweeteners after combustion and inhalation in

---

44. A metabolite is a stable compound resulting from the biochemical transformation of an initial molecule by human metabolism.

smokers' bodies. Complete combustion of 0.01 mol[45] of aspartame leads to 1.62 g of water. Ethyl ethanoate remains, i.e. an acetate, which is a varnish remover and is also found in small quantities in rum. This ester is considered not dangerous by the FDA, it is used as a flavoring agent or to decaffeinate coffee, but those who "sniff" it, are looking for a feeling of intoxication that can damage their brain.

Does it make you want to quit smoking? Many lozenges or gums are full of aspartame. Nicotinell does not hide it. The laboratory Novartis reassures on its site: "Nicotinell pastilles to suck contains aspartame (sweetener) and is therefore suitable for diabetics. For the brand Nicorette[46], there are many things in this tobacco substitute in gum, but no aspartame. In the Niquitin chewable tablets, aspartame is present, but the contraindication is visible for those who suffer from phenylketonuria.

According to German Professor Siegel, the chemical compound of concern in the vapor of electronic cigarettes is formaldehyde, which could be the result of heating propylene glycol. The e-cigarettes are sold freely, "subject to further evaluation by the authorities. They contain some of the ingredients of the "zero calorie" drinks. For those who cough while smoking "for fake", it is proposed on the Internet, additional aspartame for a better inhalation without expectoration. This is a new market, not a work of public health. Sugar like aspartame prevents coughing. Certainly, the products of electronic cigarettes do not contain polonium and do not deposit tar in the bronchial tubes, but they contain glycol, glycerine, ethanol and food flavors. What would your doctor say if you asked him: "Doctor, what is aspartyl-phenylalanine methyl ester? And what does it do in the presence of ethyl acetate?"

---

45. Mol or mole: counting unit. A mole of atoms contains about 6.02214040×1023 atoms.

46. Excipients found: amyl acetate, ethyl acetate, starch, flavor, sodium bicarbonate, butylhydroxytoluene, butyrate, ethyl butyrate, calcium carbonate, cineole, wax, carnauba wax, ethanol, eucalyptus oil, eugenol, smoker's aroma, glycerol, glycerol monostearate, gum arabic, gum base, gum dreyco, haverstroo aroma, hydrogenated vegetable oil, hypromellose, quinoline yellow, quinoline yellow aluminium lake, levomenthol, mint essence, menthol, orange essence, light magnesium oxide, polyethylene, polysorbate 80, polyvinyl acetate, potassium acesulfame, propionate, sandalwood, sodium, sorbitol, crystallized sorbitol, sucralose, orange terpenes, titanium dioxide, tutti frutti flavor, vanillin, xylitol.

Aspartame's clever name is *asparphenylamethanol* or *estermethyldasparlalanine*. With such a patronymic, it would not have inspired any confidence, added to the so-called wellness drinks. A few reminders of miscellaneous events: in December 2016, in Russia people drank "liquids unsuitable for consumption" and 49 died in Irkutsk because of methanol. In September, in Ukraine, 58 for the same reasons. In 2015 in Nigeria, people drank methanol gin, 70 died, others went blind. But who is blind today? Many blind of the facts, like methanol acidosis. In order to reassure us, health is intertwined with aspartame. For example, Coca-Cola and Sanofi have teamed up to launch Beautific Oenobiol, the fruit-enriched drink for "more beautiful beauty"! "Beautific® Oenobiol® Energy + is a non-carbonated energy drink with natural mineral water, fruit, sugar and sweeteners," it reads. It also contained acesulfame-K. Four flavors were tested in pharmacies in February 2013, drinks for hair regrowth or to regain beautiful skin and energy, and all contained E951. A few months later, the products mentioned above mentioned only sugar in the ads. Could the excipients have changed? Some Beautific are also slimming activators thanks to the glucomanan[47] E425. However, it should be known that almost all diet drinks are more or less addictive, so what are Sanofi and Coke doing together? Is the pharmaceutical laboratory only looking for profitability in diet hydration and under the benevolent protection of pharmacists? This whole universe of the "recovered line" uses the rhetoric of AminoSweet, or that of Ajinomoto: "Aspartame plays a role in the diet of diabetics, and it does not increase glucose or insulin levels in the blood." Many physicians confirm this definitive statement and verbally prescribe aspartame, confident that they are relaying the right information. "It is more difficult to disintegrate a belief than an atom," said Albert Einstein. And according to Arthur M. Evangelista, a former FDA researcher, aspartame is part of a lie to be disintegrated. His book starts from the discovery of

---

47. Because of the risk of choking, the use of E425 konjac in jelly confectionery was banned in the European Union by a directive of 18 June 2003. One may wonder why this product is accepted in pharmacies. There would be a benefit/risk for hypertension. But glucomanan, which is a fiber, absorbs substances in the stomach and intestine. Taking it together with medication can reduce the quantity and effectiveness of the medication.

Dr. Robert Mazer and James Schlatter who were looking for an inhibitor of gastrointestinal hormone secretion for an ulcer drug: the famous *aspartylphenylalanine-methyl-ester*. To believe that the dipeptide aspartame was not likely to be toxic to an early researcher is for Arthur M. Evangelista a kind of aberration. Aspartame was originally synthesized for those who suffered from an excess of a stomach hormone. In reality, a specific drug has been distributed for years to a population that knew satiety thanks to natural hunger regulators, but this "drug" causes overweight and it is aspartame.

2 - SWEETENERS, A MATTER OF TASTE: THE GOOD AND THE BAD

It's all a matter of taste and as Fénelon said before the invention of taste additives: "Foods that flatter the taste too much and that make people eat beyond their needs poison instead of nourish...".

Children reject what they don't like and become familiar with certain flavors at an early age. Five of them allow to recognize nutrients or to serve as a warning signal in case of ingestion of spoiled food containing harmful substances. The umami allows us to recognize the amino acids that make up proteins, the salty taste detects minerals including salt, the sweet taste allows us to identify nutrients rich in energy necessary for the functioning of our muscles and our brain. The perception of sweetness is linked to signals from specific receptor proteins. The sensation of pleasure that this brings is observable from birth and the industrialists are strongly interested in the olfactory receptors. Intense sweeteners are often associated with taste enhancers, additives numbered from E620 to E641. Some manufacturers add them to their products: thus these "maskers" or taste stuffers lure the brain from childhood. A form of chemical culture gradually transforms the taste choice of very young consumers. There are proteins with a sweet taste called thaumatins, of which aspartic acid is a part, such as E957 thaumatin, which is three thousand times sweeter than sugar. However, our inclination is favored by the real as well as by the false sweet taste, synonymous with energy, reward and pleasure. Acquired habits lead to overweight in sugar addicts as in sweetener addicts. How is this possible? There are neuromediators linked to synapses that activate the perception of sweeteners and make the brain believe that it can expect an energy boost. Aspartame is therefore a false sweetener trap. If the frequent use of aspartame is considered an answer to overweight and obesity, one wonders why. Strangely enough, obesity has increased at the same time as the consumption of sweeteners. Guy Fagherazzi, researcher at Inserm and lead author of a study on the subject, expressed himself as follows in an article by Erwan Lecomte of *Sciences et Avenir* in 2013: "For the same amount, the risk of developing diabetes is higher when consuming diet drinks than sweetened drinks. Women who consume one bottle per week of diet drink have a 60% higher risk of developing diabetes than women who consume the same amount of "classic" sugary drinks."

Replacing sugar with aspartame should make an overweight person melt. Toxicologist Jean-François Narbonne, whom we interviewed, notes the opposite, and cites Birch's work: "They revealed that children preferred flavors associated with caloric intake, suggesting that sweetness in itself was not sufficient to elicit food preferences, and that energy density could be the determinant of food preferences. Interactions between sweeteners and eating behavior are mediated by regulatory processes at the brain level and the neurological pathway is one of the credible hypotheses explored by several research teams. Intense sweeteners are often linked to diabetes. The incidence of the twin diseases of obesity and type 2 diabetes continues to rise in industrialized countries. Approximately two-thirds of American adults are overweight or obese with an associated risk of type 2 diabetes, cardiovascular disease and cancer. Thus, sweeteners are, on the one hand, prescribed as part of diets for diabetics, but are also, on the other hand, consumed by the general population as part of the supposed prevention of obesity and type 2 diabetes, often associated. The link between the consumption of sweetened beverages and the risk of developing type 2 diabetes was studied in 66,118 women of the Mutuelle générale de l'Éducation nationale cohort followed for 14 years. The results show that women who consume sweetened beverages have a greater consumption (+75%) than those who consume sweetened beverages. For an equal amount consumed, the risk of diabetes is higher for sweetened drinks than for sugar-sweetened drinks. On the other hand, no association with diabetes risk was found for the consumption of 100% fruit juice drinks. The question is therefore whether sweeteners do not maintain a sweetened food environment that can alter the regulation of appetite and ultimately cause energy intake. Animal studies suggest that high levels of sweetened foods induce weight gain via changes in appetite control leading to changes in eating behavior and preferences."

Regarding stevia, Professor Narbonne notes on the other hand positive effects on blood sugar and insulin levels in humans. Following the light on the trail resembles a police chase. What is most intriguing is that no one thinks of recommending another natural and safe sweetener. In addition to stevia, there is a fake sugar in this colossal market of sweeteners, a real panacea for diabetics: tagatose. This natural product does not belong to any trust and it has no impact on blood sugar levels and does not cause addiction. Why is it impossible to find in pharmacies? Because it is natural. It is found in artificial form in some diet products. Some industrial groups produce synthetic tagatose and PepsiCo has filed a patent for the use of D-tagatose in beverages and dietary products. This indicates that Pepsi seems to abandon aspartame, without communicating on the subject... The use of D-tagatose, we owe it to Pr Gilbert V. Levine, (the NASA engineer who discovered micro-organisms on Mars) under the name of tagatose or hexose, 92% as sweet as real sugar and without real caloric contribution. On April 11, 2001, this product had even obtained the status of GRAS (*Generally Recognized As Safe*), in other words recognized as healthy by the famous FDA. Tagatose is naturally present in dairy products. It can be heated without risk. The FAO and WHO have recognized it as a sweetener good for food service, but it is aspartame that is used. Why is this? Tagatose could become the flagship of a French, Swiss or European dairy industry, but only Belgium has taken over the production in the world. There is also xylitol, which is found in many fruits and vegetables, and which has the taste of sugar without the drawbacks. It is not widely used, probably because after a few months of consumption of xylitol, resistant bacteria can appear and it becomes carminative... Carminative being the elegant synonym of "which causes flatulence", in other words farts. If there is a lack of natural sweeteners available, aspartame can be found where it is not expected: in some energy drinks, doping drinks, for hyperactive people, for those who want to party and go to bed at dawn or go to work. A new market is born. The man who jumped from the highest point in the sky was sponsored by a brand of hypertonic drink. Is it healthy to couple aspartame with taurine, glucuronolactone[48] and caffeine? When you're working out hard, you need calories, otherwise you'll crash. It seems unthinkable to find aspartame in place of sugar in such sports drinks! However, some drinkers of light energy drinks end up in the emergency room; after having been boosted, they are on the floor. Are we free of our actions if we are not well informed? Can we treat someone well if we ignore the risks linked to a lifestyle based on deceptive and doping chemistry? We remember Felix Baumgartner, intrepid celestial hero, offered as a media icon to viewers who were thrilled by his audacity. At nearly 40,000 km from the ground, he jumped into the void! A sponsored human spacecraft, he broke the sound barrier before the astonished eyes of the whole world and nobody found fault with this free publicity for a space man-sandwich in the middle of the television news. It was a stunt for an industrialist who only has two products to sell: Red Bull with or without carbohydrates. The "red bull" gives "wings" even to racing cars, but we are not machines with a team of soigneurs by our side... The normal Red Bull contains[49] of "fuel", enough to last before collapsing from fatigue, but it is in the "sugar-free" that the fatal duo is nestled: acesulfame potassium and aspartame: Red Bull Sugarfree. According to Gérard Dime, a biologist at the Institute of Sports Medicine in Troyes, with Red Bull light drinks, the body is stimulated by the absorption of vitamins, taurine and caffeine. Without sugar, therefore calories, the consumer must draw his energy from his own reserves... But half of young people in France start their day without breakfast. Thirty calories

---

48. Artificial glucuronolactone can be found in other drinks such as Burn and Monster Energy.

49. Red Bull contains acesulfame-K, in addition to vitamins and dopants, glucuronolactone, which has the reputation of fighting fatigue and bringing a feeling of well-being, and is not suspected of anything except kidney toxicity, inositol, citrates, dyes and flavors. In the carbonated water of the "magic" drink, we also find ordinary caramel, E129, an acidity regulator: E331, acidifiers: citric acid, sodium citrate, theobromine with effects quite similar to those of caffeine and a preservative, potassium sorbate: E201.

per liter, is it reasonable in an energy drink? For the record, here is the text of the manufacturer: "Red Bull Sugarfree is Red Bull, but without sugar, with only three calories per 100 ml. Like Red Bull Energy Drink, Red Bull Sugarfree is a drink specially formulated for periods of activity, it invigorates the body and mind, without sugar. Red Bull Sugarfree gives wings in all circumstances, whether at work, while studying, playing video games, sports, on the road, with friends at home or out. In short, Red Bull Sugarfree is for everyone who combines an active lifestyle with a zest for life[50].

Seen in this light, it makes you want to try it, but Australian doctors have expressed concern about the ravages of this kind of low-fat stimulant, as it can cause cardiovascular disease and sometimes death. Scott Willoughby, from the Cardiovascular Research Center in Adelaide, explains that after an hour, sugar-free Red Bull makes the cardiovascular system abnormal. Consuming energy drinks from two cans per day multiplies the risks for the heart (palpitations and tachycardia). This is the result of an Australian study, published in the *International Journal of Cardiology*, conducted among patients aged 13 to 40 years, admitted to the emergency room of Lyell McEwin Hospital between 2014 and 2015 for heart palpitations. The products contained thicken the blood. Dopants united with aspartame are also found in Monster Light. What do aspartame and all the components of an energy drink together, with or without alcohol, with or without medication, with or without drugs? What are the harmful interactions and who can answer? Why are we being led to believe that this is a controversy? Isn't it finally the best way to hide scientific truths that are difficult to grasp by the common man? Then time bombs are on sale. Vodka-Red Bull is the cocktail of nightclubs, but also Monster, Dark Dog, Burn, Frelon Detox and so many others. The "Health" supplement of the newspaper *Le Monde* reported on *rave parties* in 2012 and Dr. Laurent Chevallier, nutritionist, member of the Réseau Environnement Santé (RES) wondered then: "How many accidents will it take to make decisions?" ANSES reported six reports of serious adverse effects (epilepsy, coma, tremor, anxiety). ANSES reported 30 cases of cardiological problems, including two recent fatal

---

50. This text can be found on the Redbull.fr website.

2 - Sweeteners, a matter of taste: the good and the bad

cases, epileptic seizures or psychiatric disorders, often following the consumption of boosted alcohol, a term used by young people. For a long time, Red Bull's boss had students (*student brand managers)* recruited on campuses, in charge of organizing parties where Red Bull was initially provided free of charge. The DJs were pampered by *Herr* Dietrich Mateschitz's sales staff, who did not forget to leave empty cans in the toilets of the establishments to give visitors the impression that some customers came there to take their "shot" (*Les Echos*, 2012). Surfers and other sportsmen have become addicted. When Red Bull Sugarfree makes proven deaths, there will be someone to say that the drink is not good for all ages and all hours, and that sugar-free does not prevent anyone from seeking calories elsewhere! It seems to be accepted that you can drink energy drinks without sugar and the contraindications are obvious. Where would the energy without calories come from? The manufacturer of Red Bull that we contacted by mail, declared us via its press officer, that the group communicated only on the sporting events and not on the consequences of the light in health. About 40 million liters of these energy drinks are consumed each year in France. So two official deaths would be nothing? There are risks of heart attack and stroke by blood clots. According to the journalist Marie Huppé the death of two members of the national squash team of Kuwait would be due to the regular consumption of an energy drink...

Aspartame is frequently used with other chemical substances, in Europe 30,000 can be used and some mixtures can be disastrous! The exposure routes are multiple: food and drugs, but the medical profession is unaware of what aspartame, neotame, additives, residues of pesticide or veterinary treatments, in the same human body... Doctors have not had any explanation on the effects of the dissolution of sweeteners in remains called metabolites that can accumulate especially in the brain. How many food and drug additives over the years disrupt our metabolism[51]? The whole of the molecular transformations which take place in an uninterrupted way in our cells so that our organism is at its best can be disturbed. E951 is found in some

---

51. Metabolism, from the Greek *meta*: "succession", "transformation", and *bolein*: "action of throwing".

medicines because of its sweetness and its role as a preservative. E951 can be a deadly poison. Anti-epileptic drugs may contain aspartame or may not mention that they should not be combined with aspartame because it contributes to seizures which contribute to the drugs, which cause more seizures... Hellish chain! Really, the doctors who take care of us should be more interested in toxicology in order to prescribe safe remedies in conscience. New rare diseases, sometimes called emerging diseases, are multiplying and aspartame seems to be one of their promoters. It's a bit like a lottery. Some people will have no problem, others will suffer. Some will come across aspartame made by pharmaceutical laboratories, others will swallow something *made in* China. The aspartame powder arrives in a can and the manufacturers promise that they add a little arsenic for shipping to avoid the humidity that aspartame is so afraid of! And will we find aspartame in baby bottles to accustom infants? It is already done in the United States in what is called *baby food*! Children are more vulnerable than adults and the effects of methanol on fetuses and babies should not worry any mother... On the French site santémagazine.fr, to the question: "Can we give sweeteners to our children?" The answer is: "In reasonable amounts, aspartame is not toxic." On this site, the toxic dose would be 30 cans light/day according to Pr Patrick Tounian and EFSA. Pr Tounian adds that sweeteners are good for making small obese patients lose weight. The article gives, however, the opposite opinion of Professor Laurent Chevallier.

The freedom of consumption allows almost everything to be bought on the Internet and everything that constitutes aspartame is for sale: phenylalanine, for example. But then, there are informative warnings[52]. So phenylalanine alone would be an appetite suppressant,

---

52. "L-phenylalanine is an essential amino acid that the body cannot synthesize and must be supplied by the diet. It is the precursor of the neurotransmitters norepinephrine (cerebral equivalent of adrenaline), epinephrine and dopamine (which contributes to the feeling of well-being), as well as L-tyrosine: a light and well-tolerated cerebral stimulant. Through other pathways, it can also be converted to phenylethylamine, a naturally occurring substance in the brain, which positively influences mood. L-phenylalanine also triggers the production of the hormone cholecystokinin (CCK) in the gut, which gives the brain a satiety signal, thus calming the appetite. In humans, the administration half an hour before a meal of a mixture of amino acids - including Lphenylalanine - causes a 22.5% decrease in food consumption: it is a natural and safe appetite suppressant.

2 - Sweeteners, a matter of taste: the good and the bad

while aspartame would increase the appetite? This amino acid is commercially available to promote fat burning. According to the advertisements of the parapharmacy, it would stimulate the nervous influx between the neurons. Phenylalanine is primarily a transmitter, and here is what the Equi-Nutri brand says about it:

"L-phenylalanine calms bulimia and cravings for sweets by producing the hormone cholecystokinin (CCK) in the intestine, which gives the brain a signal to feel full, thus calming the appetite. Avoid in case of high blood pressure or anxiety attacks. Keep out of reach of children. Other contraindications: pregnant and breast-feeding women, high blood pressure, diabetes and phenylketonuria, taking an MAOI antidepressant." Why don't health agencies mention this kind of information? Because it should be explained that CKK[53] is a peptide hormone secreted by the mucosa of the duodenum, returned to the bloodstream and that it causes the release of enzymes by the pancreas and increases bile, that CKK plays a role in satiety and can develop tolerance to morphine. Perhaps CKK is what the chemical engineer Schlatter was trying to master? Phenylalanine as a dietary supplement is accompanied by this statement: "Not to be taken during pregnancy unless directed by a therapist. Store away from a source of heat, light or moisture." The parapharmacy of self-medication is getting covered!

It was my pharmacist who alerted me to the fact that diet drinks expire quickly, and that this is the best before date. In general, diet products do not keep well. Coca-Cola specifies on one of its sites that after this date, "the product may no longer meet the high quality standards". But when there is aspartame that we know is unstable, nothing is specified. As for the Red Bull light that can be bought on the Internet, the only mention is: "Please always read the warning labels and indications provided before using or consuming the product." On the site Red Bull zero calories and zero sugar: nothing is reported either on the expiration dates ... Just the usual refrain: aspartame is one of the most tested sugar substitutes in the world ... It happens that supermarkets get rid of expired batches by

---

53. Cholecystokinin is a polypeptide. Its gene is located on the human chromosome 3. It is interrupted by too much gastric acidity.

selling them. No one to tell us what happens to these cocktails of expired substances mixed with possibly degraded aspartame...

In addition to the regulatory bodies of 134 countries, experts from the World Health Organization (WHO), the Food and Agriculture Organization of the United Nations (FAO) and the European Commission's Scientific Committee on Food (SCF) have studied aspartame and concluded that it is safe. To understand the risks induced for some, we must go beyond the fact that aspartame is a food ingredient made from two amino acids. It is known that it is rapidly transformed when heated. But how do its compounds get eliminated in the body and in how long? It is only reported that beverages containing E951 should be kept away from heat (same thing for medicines). But the body is not a refrigerator!

3 - What is aspartame?

Let's take a closer look. E951 is made of phenylalanine (50%), aspartic acid (40%), and methyl ester (10%), which turns into methyl alcohol - or methanol - after ingestion and into diketopiperazine and other neurotoxic and carcinogenic products resulting from its breakdown. Diketopiperazine is considered a drug[54], but derived from aspartame or neotame, no law prevents its ingestion.

Induced **methanol** is a central nervous system depressant. At room temperature, it is a liquid solvent used as an antifreeze, fuel, and *ethyl* alcohol denaturant. Aspartame at the "right temperature", when ingested, produces methanol at very low doses, but it is the same methanol, harmful in cans, the same one used in Formula 1 racing or added to wastewater in sewage plants to feed the bacteria that will transform nitrates into nitrogen. Although the amounts involved are very small, no one would ever think of sipping a few drops of racing fuel to feel "lighter". The chemical methanol is toxic

---

54. According to the French Health Security Agency, the main impurity of aspartame comes from the famous diketopiperazine also called dioxopiperazine. DROGUE INFO SERVICE mentions piperazine - often mixed with cocaine, ecstasy and amphetamines - as a drug, it causes uncontrolled movements, psychosis, hallucinations, paranoia, etc. DROGUE INFO SERVICE states: "Piperazines come in several forms: powder, capsule, tablet and liquid. Legal status: in France, BZP (benzylpiperazine) is classified as a narcotic. Its use is forbidden: article L. 3421-1 of the Public Health Code provides for fines (3 750 €) and prison sentences (up to one year). Incitement to use and trafficking and the presentation of the product in a favorable light are prohibited: article L 3421-4 of the Public Health Code provides for fines (up to 75 000 €) and prison sentences (up to 5 years). Acts of trafficking are prohibited: Articles 222-34 to 222-43 of the Penal Code provide for fines (up to €7,500,000) accompanied by prison sentences (up to thirty years of criminal imprisonment)."

by ingestion, inhalation and skin absorption. The industries that manufacture it know that it can be lethal and that in "non-lethal doses" it causes a decrease or complete loss of vision, accompanied by acidosis (abnormal acidity of the plasma). Some of these symptoms are found in aspartame addicts. Comparison is not reason, but zero precaution offers a zero guarantee. In the industry, methanol requires a DANGER label. This liquid is highly toxic if swallowed, corrosive and mutagenic and can cause genetic defects.

This alcohol is a hydrocarbon miscible with water[55]. And if it is biodegradable in water, is it in the blood? In forensic medicine, methanol is said to be very well resorbed, whether by digestive, pulmonary or cutaneous routes[56]. Methanol intoxication in drunks is detected by the presence of formic acid in the blood serum.

Formaldehyde from methanol is used as a food formaldehyde or for the preservation of silage at a concentration of about 30% with 1 to 5% methanol. This formaldehyde is also called methanal or formaldehyde. Formaldehyde is used as a fungicide, antimicrobial and disinfectant. It preserves and decontaminates in industrial use. But would we consume it with our eyes closed? The oral dose of 10 to 100 ml of formalin is considered fatal in humans. Fortunately, we are far from it with a light in our hands! But we ingest it without knowing it. Formaldehyde residues are found in milk and it is used as a preservative in skimmed milk for pigs, under the name E240. Cattle and pigs that have eaten cake all year long are soaked in it, and this poison, even at low doses, is added to that of our star drinks. According to *La Documentation française*: "The only available data on the acute toxicity of formaldehyde in livestock are based on observations of breeding practices made by veterinarians, but the doses could not be precisely determined."

The use of formaldehyde is varied: it is used as a disinfectant, fixative, preservative of cadavers or vaccines, it treats warts, it allows to fill the canals of devitalized teeth, to embalm the bodies, to produce

---

55. Methanol biodegrades readily in water and soil. At high concentrations (greater than 1%) in fresh or salt water, it can adversely affect aquatic life in the immediate vicinity of the spill.

56. 70 to 80% are metabolized by the liver to formaldehyde and then to formic acid, part of which is transformed into CO_2. Methanol is eliminated in the exhaled air as unchanged or as CO_2 (10-30%) and in the urine as methanol (less than 10%) or formic acid.

polymers, to glue tapestries, to preserve food, to agriculture... It is also a corrosion inhibitor in the extraction of shale gas. It is used in the manufacture of paints and explosives. Several European countries limit or prohibit its use. Officially, it has no side effects at usable doses, but there are no long-term studies, nor on cocktail effects with other toxic additives. The import of formaldehyde-treated products is subject to regulation or ban, and several European countries ban formaldehyde-treated products. A European bill sets thresholds not to be exceeded in food for this biocide (i.e. life-killing) product.

A small health summary is necessary. According to EFSA experts, formaldehyde is rapidly metabolized. But this tissue fixative in anatomy laboratories is classified by the INRS and other organizations as a carcinogen.

Aspartic acid and **phenylalanine** are both neurotoxic. As we now know, E951 is transformed in our body from about 30°C. However, unless we are dead, every human being remains at an average temperature of 37°C and there is always incompatibility between a vital organ and what weakens or damages it.

Formic acid, the last degradation of aspartame, is used in the textile or leather industry and is used in the formulation of insecticides, lacquers, solvents and household products as a substitute for mineral acids. In a diluted state, it is used in human food as a food additive, under the name E236. It is used as a preservative and antibacterial agent in livestock feed. The icing on the cake, it is used in poultry farming to eradicate E. coli (*Escherichia coli*, fecal bacilli) from which aspartame is derived in its manufacture. As for beekeepers, they use it as an acaricide.

In its 1975 report, the WHO referred to certain additives and their breakdowns, *and* the committee officially considered that at this early stage of toxicological evaluation, **the diketopiperazine** from the aspartame manufacturing process was 5%.

Now let's get to the process of making aspartame. It requires a cloned fecal bacterium to be created, one that also makes life-saving insulin. Monsanto discovered that by genetically modifying a certainly bovine bacterium, phenylalanine would be made faster. In the report published by *The Independent*, Monsanto openly admitted that their modified bacteria was a key step in the process of creating aspartame: "We have two varieties of bacteria, one is conventionally modified, and the other is genetically modified. It has a modified enzyme. It has a different amino acid."

For the record, Monsanto was working on growth hormone from E. coli. A mutant strain was first spotted in the United States in 1994. *Escherichia coli* is an intestinal bacterium that looks like a sausage under the microscope (fecal coliform) and its cell division takes place every twenty minutes. Some E. coli are non-pathogenic, others are hemorrhagic. GMO E. coli are very valuable to the industry as small factories for industrial and medical products, they produce what is required of them, in this case aspartame. When all the factors are in place for the bacteria to grow and gorge themselves on carbonaceous food, alcohol, nitrogen, urea, glucose, etc., before moving on to the fermentation phase, they produce amino acids (a bit like in sewage plants), and they gobble it all up. Ammonia water can be added to their permanent lunch and when there are enough amino acids, the contents of the fermentation go to the centrifuge which separates the elements. The amino acids are pumped and crystallized, dried for the synthesis phase. In general, phenylalanine is modified by reaction with methanol, acetic acid. Then, it is the purification stage, the solvent is dissolved in aqueous ethanol. The source of this explanation is reliable: it comes directly from NutraSweet.

To manufacture L-aspartic acid and L-phenylalanine, genetically modified E. coli are used, which are the best workers in the world and do not require wages or breaks... These Stakhanovists are real miniature production bombs! The work of Y. Chao, T. Lo and N. Luo are edifying: *Aspartase-hyperproducing mutants of Escherichia coli B.* Those of N. Nishimura and M. Kisumi explain the advantage of adding glucose and nitrogen in the food of these mutant "bugs"[57] which produce a lot for the industry.

Let's go back to the components of aspartame to try to understand what is "wrong" with what we are told and what we are not told:

___

57. The thesis of Dr. Ziad el-Hajj, a post-doctoral fellow in the Department of Biology in Montreal, reports the isolation of a mutant *Escherichia coli that is* seven hundred and fifty times larger than normal, but cannot divide (January 27, 2012).

Phenylalanine is an amino acid normally found in the brain and supplied by the diet, but by ingesting aspartame, too much phenylalanine in the brain and blood can occur. Neurosurgeon Russell Blaylock says that excessive levels of phenylalanine can cause schizophrenia and stroke.

Aspartic acid is an amino acid that in its free form causes an increase in neurotransmitters in certain areas of the brain. In normal circumstances, they facilitate the transmission of information between neurons. In excess, they destroy some of them by allowing the invasion of calcium in overdose, which triggers an excessive increase of free radicals that kill nerve cells and create holes in the brain. But at least 75% of the nerve cells in an area of the brain must be killed before a chronic disease such as multiple sclerosis, Alzheimer's or Parkinson's can be detected.

Methanol degrades on heating into **formaldehyde and formic acid**. It causes numerous neurological disorders.

Formaldehyde is neurotoxic, carcinogenic, and interferes with DNA reproduction, alters the retina and causes prenatal malformations.

DKP is a product derived from phenylalanine which is implicated, among other things, in the development of brain tumors and causes changes in cholesterol levels according to American toxicologist Jacqueline Verrett. DKP is synthesized in drinks containing aspartame after prolonged storage.

If aspartame is made from GMO E. coli bacteria, we must focus on the bacteria of our own intestinal flora which are linked to our health. The intestinal flora forms an ecosystem which the richer it is, the better it promotes health. Those who are the fattest are often the poorest in intestinal flora. Light eaters suffer from poor intestinal flora, which is another factor that makes them fatter and more vulnerable! It is in the United States that we find the most malnourished obese people. Digestive bacteria vary according to our diet and lifestyle. They should protect us and participate in the immune system, but it is a vicious circle when the light degrades the microbiota. This sweetener, "good for the figure, good for the form", promotes and accelerates dysfunctions!

In conclusion of this chapter, sweeteners would be diabetogenic through the microbiota. Here is a sentence that I could never have written or understood before this investigation. I hope it is the same for you, reader.

According to Dr. Isabelle Catala: "It is important to know that most of these sweeteners pass through the digestive tract without being digested and that they therefore arrive without any modification in contact with the intestinal flora, which is essential for proper physiological functioning. We know that the type of diet of a slim and healthy person, as well as that of a diabetic or overweight person, will condition the nature and functioning of the microbiota. And conversely, alterations in the microbiota have been associated with an increased risk of metabolic syndrome."

CQFD, right? But how do we come to destroy our intestinal flora? By choices that are sometimes teleguided by flourishing and appetizing advertisements.

4 - Aspartame promotes diabetes and neurological disorders

It all starts in our shopping cart. As you shop, candy with childhood-colored packaging catches your eye, but it's full of E202 and E211. *Trust the* packaging seems to say: it's *for kids.* The point of sale is not there to educate you and the cashier is not a toxicologist and does not know that E202 is potassium sorbate, that E211 is sodium benzoate which can cause hyperactivity syndrome when combined with dyes. E211 would cause allergies in the presence of vitamin C, and it would be transformed into benzene... However, this sweetener is found in Fanta, Oasis, Pepsi Max, Sprite, Nestea and Diet Coke itself loaded with acesulfame-K and aspartame... By buying a pack of Diet Coke, one is actually looking at the history of the falsified taste, of aspartame and its industrial, pharmaceutical, political and financial implications. But the incriminating substances have all been approved for human consumption by European food experts. The book should therefore end there.

However, aspartame seems to be the promoter of certain diseases including diabetes. There are countries where half the population is overweight. It is therefore necessary to know what precisely is attributable to sugar or aspartame, to understand the link with type 2 diabetes and what it causes in turn as a disease. The chemical and disruptive light is a false answer that is beginning to ruin public and private health insurance.

Those who want to keep their figure, who, instead of eating and drinking healthily, bet on zero calories and sweeteners, make a fatal mistake. The absence of carbohydrates causes hypoglycemia, which leads to a craving for sugars. It's a vicious cycle. So, if sweeteners are useless, why make them aids that ultimately disrupt the metabolism, deceive and alter our brain? But in fact, why did we make war on sugar? The act of "medicalizing" diet as Jean-François Narbonne explains it, was done in a supposed concern of form and health for others. Professor in toxicology, he was approached as an expert by Coca-Cola to give his opinion on aspartame in its drinks:

"Due to globalization and the resulting Marrakech Accords in 1995, the responsibility of company managers has changed, particularly in France. Thus, the company manager must not only comply with regulations but also ensure the safety of products, taking into account all the progress of technical and scientific knowledge available. To guarantee this multiple information, managers obviously do not go to meetings, symposiums, and seminars, or delve into scientific and technical literature. One of the solutions adopted at the time by the major food and distribution groups was to create "information and advisory committees" made up of experts covering the various disciplines concerned (doctors, microbiologists, veterinarians, toxicologists, nutritionists, technologists, chemical analysts) who could provide up-to-date information for crisis prevention. In view of the shortage of experts in food toxicology in France, I was asked to participate in several information committees. On several occasions, I was asked to give an update on the evolution of the aspartame dossier and new sweeteners such as stevia. It was during one of these committees for a large soda group established in France that I explained, more than ten years ago, that the future of aspartame was darkening, that suspicions about its harmlessness were mounting and that the promotion of diet sodas was based on a nutritional deception that contributed to the addiction to this substance, leading to the consumption of other sweetened foods. I advised them to eventually look at other sweeteners such as stevia extracts for their diet range, which they felt was unavoidable. This very advanced position at the time led to the end of my collaboration, as they were preparing the launch of their zero range."

And why so many diet or sugary drinks rather than just spring water? It is obvious, there is no addiction to water. If water has never killed anyone, unless it is too high in salt and is given to elderly people with high blood pressure, why are there so many drinks saturated with sweeteners? Are tumors, diabetes and other diseases related to aspartame?

In France, the French Agency for Food Safety (AFSSA) had officially raised the question of a possible link between exposure to aspartame and brain tumors in a May 2002 file. The AFSSA had been seized on October 16, 2000 by the General Directorate of Competition, Consumption and Fraud Control on this link. The file exposed a possible risk for the public health, to conclude at the end that the hypotheses were alarmist. "In conclusion, AFSSA considers that the current state of scientific data does not allow to establish a relationship between exposure to aspartame and brain tumors in humans or animals.

This text was signed by Martin Hirsch. Diabetologists are serene. But then where would certain brain abnormalities come from?

We asked Professor Narbonne what he thought about the interaction between glutamate and aspartame. He answered that at the brain level, it was the greatest risk. While the answer is complex, it seems to be clear-cut. And here are the excitotoxins accused again:

"Dye/glutamate and dye/aspartame combinations induce neurotoxicity by a factor of 4 and 7 respectively. The loss of nerve cells that can be caused by glutamate and aspartame in excess is the reason why they are called "excitotoxins". They "excite" or stimulate nerve cell death by allowing excessive calcium invasion. This invasion triggers excessive levels of free radicals that kill the cells. Excitotoxicity is a pathological process of neuronal damage and destruction by hyperactivation of excitatory neurotransmitters. Glutamate acts as a neurotransmitter facilitating the transmission of information between neurons; and depending on the dose, neurological disorders can be observed. In young people, the hypothalamus and hippocampus are affected, and in adults, skeletal development, obesity, and sterility are affected. Neurological signs can also be Huntington's disease, an orphan disease that results in neurological degeneration, acquired immunodeficiency syndrome, attack of retinal neurons, headaches, and what is called "Chinese restaurant syndrome", the one that is triggered in less than a quarter of an hour after starting his meal and is linked to the additive E621, glutamate. A possible interaction between glutamate and aspartame was demonstrated in vitro in 2005 and even in vivo in mice in 2006. In order to highlight possible interactions between authorized and separately evaluated food additives, the neurotoxic effects of four additives were studied in binary combinations. These were brilliant blue (E133) and L-glutamic acid (E621), and quinoline yellow (E104) and aspartame (E951). Mouse neuroblastoma cells[58] NB2a are put in the presence of the additives, and the induction of growth and differentiation of young neurons is studied. After 24 hours, the cells are fixed and stained, the length of the neurons is measured by microscopy and subjected to image analysis. The estimated neurotoxicity by inhibition of neuron growth increases by 10 to 50% with azo dyes and by 50 to 60% with aspartame or glutamate."

These complex but effective studies could, according to Prof. Narbonne, explain the neurotoxic effects of aspartame with the appearance of attention deficit and hyperactivity syndrome (ADHD) in children with a high level of aspartame consumption. He also points to a study by the American Academy of Neurology, published in 2013, which exposes the effects due to regular intake of sweeteners: 293,925 people, aged 50 to 71, took part. From 1995 to 1996, the researchers evaluated the consumption of beverages such as soft drinks, teas, fruit cocktails and coffee. About ten years later, the experts checked which participants had had a nervous breakdown since the year 2000. By comparing the consumption of the 11,311 participants who had been diagnosed with depression with those who had not, they found that those who consumed more than four cans of sweetened soft drinks per day were unfortunately 30% more likely to develop depression than those who did not consume them. On the other hand, those who consume four or more coffees per day would see their risk decrease by 10% compared to those who do not consume them. In conclusion, the risk of depression is increased when the product is "aspartame". New accusation and new silence. The precautionary principle only interests consumers for the moment...

---

58. Neuroblastoma is the most common extra-cranial solid tumor in young children. It is a cancer involving embryonic stem cells of the neural crest that constitutes the sympathetic autonomic nervous system. Neuroblastoma can be associated with Hirschprung's disease, which is an abnormality of the terminal part of the intestine causing obstructions.

5 - WHO TO BELIEVE?

Despite all the above, diabetics should not have to worry about getting seriously ill by loving to eat and drink diet. One thing is for sure: no one will get the model size via the aspartame fairy. The advertising is only seductive. Fashion artists dress up bottles and cans with their art... The very talented and media-savvy Jean-Paul Gaultier, Marc Jacobs, Karl Lagerfeld and Chantal Thomass have played the game of decorating diet drinks... And when consumers find their legal drug on the shelves, signed by a big name to charm them, they have no fear for their health. Mr. Everyman is not paranoid, he lives in a multidimensional labyrinth, constantly alerted, so this attention to him reassures him. He worships the 0% and doesn't understand why, by redoubling his efforts and purchases, he doesn't lose an ounce, worse, he puts on weight. He doesn't know how much the bill costs. He doesn't know how his body works.

To get out of the sterile questioning, we need simple and explicit answers. But since everything is unclear, the FDA can continue to say that aspartame can be heated to make desserts, while others say that cooking with E951 is criminal. Who to believe? Is it absolutely necessary to add the statement: "Beware, cooking kills slowly" before diabetologists are scientifically and intimately convinced of this? Some consumers blindly follow recipes with aspartame that are easily found on the Internet. For example, you can make a low-fat version of a flan with aspartame powder, such as this ASPARTAME PHEASTER FLAN (for five people).

- 500 ml of milk 1/2 skimmed or skimmed ;
- 4 large eggs ;
- 2 tablespoons of liquid vanilla ;
- 5 to 8 level tablespoons of powdered aspartame.
Preheat the oven thermostat 6 for ten minutes. In a bowl, beat the eggs with the liquid vanilla and sweetener, add the milk and mix. Pour the mixture into a smooth-rimmed baking dish. To cook with the furnace during one hour (source: forum of dukan.et.nous).

The link between Dukan and aspartame indicates that the former doctor is not a chemist. At normal body temperature, the metamorphosis of aspartame takes place and its metabolites can be toxic. Note that the manufacturer Ajinomoto offers the Dukan diet as part of nutritional and caloric information. In an interview published by the site auféminin.com, Dukan said that "there has never been an incident" with aspartame and added:

"My position is the same as that of many scientists and it is very clear: **aspartame is not the cause.** This controversy is the result of attacks launched by "crows" whose job it is almost. I personally have no interest in advocating aspartame, I defend it because I think so. Aspartame has been around for twenty-five years. No country has ever banned it. It is used by my estimate by at least 1 billion people around the world in the form of diet drinks, chewing gum or any other kind of product in which it is found and there has never been an incident in those twenty-five years. I don't even know of any food or medicine that has been tested for so long and on so many people! By the way, during an interview, I asked Professor Khayat (one of the first oncologists in the United States) for his opinion. I asked him the question clearly: does aspartame present a risk of cancer? His answer was just as clear: NO! As an oncologist, he was much more concerned about being overweight, which is a real cancer risk, unlike aspartame. So even insofar as aspartame can reduce overweight, it is rather recommended than not recommended!"

Not at all is not an answer. And one would like to answer that if aspartame makes you fat, one can be offended by such "lightness"! Only real pastry chefs are careful about their health. They know not to heat aspartame. Better still, at the pastry school, they explain that the law authorizes the use of aspartame, but that maltisol (E965), a polyol that does not damage the teeth and only causes gastric problems, is preferable to the use of sweeteners forbidden for infants and young children (source of 2004 for the artisanal pastry industry). We would expect the same precaution from the EFSA and the FDA!

In industrial pastry, we learn that Canderel proposed sucralose in 2009. Would there have been a withdrawal of the manufacturers of E951 for a less dangerous product? Sucralose is an intense artificial sweetener, synthesized from a selective chlorination of sucrose. It sweetens three times more than aspartame. The second strength of sucralose is that it remains stable to heat. It seems to be less harmful and less disruptive than aspartame. When consumed, it is largely evacuated naturally. Non-carcinogenic, non-mutagenic, it would not harm diabetics, would only cause bloating, intestinal, stomach and muscle pains, some diarrhea, bladder problems and at worst: a psychotic panic... All this to keep the line... *Diet, light, slim,* are English words most often synonymous with sweeteners and fitness. Christophe Charret (CEO of Diet World), a specialist in dietetics, thinks that:

"Dietetics is the study of a set of rules to govern the diet of the human being. It is not invariable because it is subject to the growth of knowledge but also to fashion effects. Its application or not has a significant impact on our daily performance and our various faculties. Therefore the question is to know if aspartame is to be catalogued around this definition as beneficial, neutral, or harmful? It is good to take this reflection with the basic principles of Asians who always ask themselves the following question in relation to food: "Will this food be harmful to me?", unlike Westerners who ask themselves the following question: "Will it be good for me? Simple nuance but a big one. In my humble opinion, if we take only the aspect of weight balance included in the notion of dietetics, aspartame is an interesting substitute since it is much less caloric than glucose. However, in the whole sense of the term dietetics, the answer is negative. First of all, because logically we cannot replace what nature offers us. The latter will offer a form of perfection for man when we have grasped the part of the mechanisms that still eludes us. The sweetening substances exist in a natural state, they are even omnipresent and so much the better for our cells which cannot do without them and make us feel any lack by the symptoms of hypoglycemia. From the moment it is scientifically established that aspartame, when exposed to a certain temperature, is transformed after several stages into formic acid, which is a dangerous poison, and that aspartame is overused by a large number of industrialists in the food industry, we have the right to be concerned and to classify it as harmful. Formaldehyde can cause many neurological disorders, in an insidious and slow way, which is why there is perhaps a lack of global awareness to start a serious reflection on this subject. Aspartame creates a compulsive need for carbohydrates in consumers. This compulsive state also leads us away from basic dietary principles.

Isn't the main thing to look for what suits our body, our metabolism best? For the moment we know one thing, aspartame is part of the chemical components of our food: something that has not happened since Neanderthal. After four hundred and fifty thousand years of non-industrial food, will our body get used to it? Are we going to pass to mithridatization, which consists in ingesting increasing doses of a toxic product, in order to acquire a kind of insensitivity or resistance to the product? We are not equal in front of our plates and Philippe Durrèche, advisor in collective catering for local authorities, had noticed that the canteens prefer light to natural:

"Some menus for children or the elderly look like time bombs. It is clear that in the name of staff comfort, food safety, and the search for the lowest price, the cooks have been replaced by "box openers". There are few fresh and organic products, but products whose pedigree is unknown. There are sweeteners in some products from the food industry. They accumulate between drinks, desserts and even some hams. And not everything that looks delicious to a child's palate is good for their health. Dyes and sweeteners are found in yoghurts and cheeses and aspartame is imposed on diabetics in retirement homes, without asking their opinion. In local authorities, day-care centers, canteens and retirement homes, menus must first meet a set of specifications established by the Ministry of the

Economy, Finance and Industry: the GEMRCN (Groupe d'étude des marchés de restauration collective et de nutrition). This famous "paving stone", which is the equivalent of a ream of paper, goes back over what is good, what must be present (to the nearest gram) and balanced for all populations. It is aimed at the insiders who are the chefs, the elected officials who are in charge of the catering of their city, the nutritionists and dieticians who intervene for the cities or the catering companies. From birth to death, the nutritional "bible" presents product family after product family. We will thus find accepted flavor enhancers, glucose-fructose syrup which has a much higher sweetening power than the classic white sugar (sucrose). One of the dangers of this syrup without vitamins and extracted from its original food, purified and presented in the form of syrup or powder, is that if our taste buds and our brain do not make the difference between the usual sugars and this last one, the body, him, quickly makes the difference and will store this surplus of fructose directly in the form of greases. The diet may therefore seem preferable. Unfortunately, blond or bleached heads consume what is more of a chemical than a nutritional nature. According to an Australian study, our children consume 100 additives per day. Then there are the chemical flavourings. Chemical synthesis has made it possible to manufacture products that do not exist in nature... If "the dose makes the poison", we can only deplore exposure to these products for our children. Even with high safety margins, how can we evaluate the real absorption of additives for each person?

The late Philippe Durrèche mentioned a video shot in a school in Australia: *Children: test tubes on legs*. Foods that seemed harmless but that contain flavor enhancers, coloring agents, sweeteners and other additives are banned, and as if by miracle, attention and behavioral disorders decrease significantly in young consumers. According to him, doctors in France, during their nutrition consultations, noticed an evolution towards a low diversity of food, and many people have monophagous tendencies, i.e. a propensity to eat a lot of the same product. For example, some people drink sodas every day, often of the same brand, and cannot "stand" drinking water, others are only used to two or three types of ready-made meals full of additives, and others always eat the same cookies, which are often of mediocre quality. This is why schools should be the first to introduce healthy, additive-free foods. Philippe Durrèche has fought for canteens without aspartame or additives and has made more and more followers by showing that it is possible, healthy and not more expensive!

Sugar or aspartame drinks are replacing water and schools often have soda machines! So there are direct and indirect sources to propel diabetes, which is affecting more and more children. The numbers speak for themselves. The evolution of diabetes in the world went from 30 million people in 1985 to 285 million in 2010 with a prospect of 435 million for 2030. In France, treatments for diabetes represented nearly 2 billion euros, twice as much as in the year 2000! Type 2 diabetes linked to diet is due to a lack of activity and an often poor and overly rich diet. Sweeteners then become gas pedals of this disease. The pancreas produces more and more inefficient insulin. According to Christian Boitard, director of the ITMO (Circulation, Metabolism, Nutrition) of the Hôtel-Dieu Hospital, one person in 15 will be affected by diabetes by 2030. The impact of canteen food in the diet and eating habits is already participating in the aggravation. However, as we can see: aspartame is part of the gustatory panoply of many canteens, and of course of the industrial nutrition found on the shelves. In addition to this, meals at home are often too energetic, sweet and aspartame-filled. Trace elements have no place in fast food. Thus obesity is on the rise. Canteens are places where weight is gained and where there is not necessarily a free water fountain! As for marketing, it will mainly focus on high-risk products. Do we have to wait for an increase in the number of obese children to be concerned about it? And what about the retirement homes that claim for the most part that aspartame has no effect on weight and health. Except on a few courageous sites such as info-retraite.fr whose homepage informs and talks about Dr. Roberts. This world expert on aspartame poisoning was a diabetic and wrote a book called *Defense Against Alzheimer's Disease* in which he explained how aspartame poisoning aggravates Alzheimer's disease. His diabetic patients had memory loss, confusion and severe visual disturbances.

The body is not prepared for chemical-based nutrition. It's not just aspartame you need to watch out for. Studies done on small rodents fed sucralose have shown that they suffered from atrophy of the thymus. This tiny organ is responsible for the proper development of the immune system in children, children who all over the world love chemical sodas... After puberty, our thymus shrivels up naturally because the natural defense system has become strong enough. The addition of harmful "E's" is dangerous to the balance of the immune system. Perhaps this is also a new lead to find the source of some autoimmune diseases? In any case, we should do without sweeteners until adulthood, do without useless sweeteners altogether, so that the digestion of food is beneficial to health! The sweet scam may one day turn out to be a health scandal. Before you make up your mind, the manufacture of aspartame itself is somewhat difficult to digest...

6 -The manufacture of aspartame in France

Some factories continue to produce it, others assemble it with other additives. The undisputed leader of aspartame remains today Ajinomoto. For Europe, this group had installed its factory in France. A journalist from *L'Usine nouvelle* predicted a real success: "The Japanese group is strengthening its aspartame production capacity in Japan and the United States. The market seemed buoyant in 2005 and here is the text of Juliette Bosse-Platière published on January 6, 2005: "World leader in aspartame with 40% of market share, Ajinomoto intends to remain so. The Japanese food group will therefore invest more than 43 million euros between now and March 2006 in its two factories in Yokkaichi, Japan, and Gravelines, dedicated to its flagship product. It will increase its production from 6,000 to 10,000 tonnes per year, and will thus be able to supply more than half the market. It will then retain its leading position ahead of the two other major manufacturers, NutraSweet, owned by the American investment fund J. W. Childs Associates, and Holland Sweetener Co (HSC), a joint venture between Japan's Tosoh and the Netherlands' DSM.

And what did the journalist Gérard Muteaud write in *Les Echos* on 7 January 1991? NutraSweet, a subsidiary of the American chemical group Monsanto, is going to join forces with the Japanese giant Ajinomoto, a biotechnology specialist, to build a plant in the Nord-Pas-de-Calais region." In the article, we learn that Brussels was preparing to impose customs duties on NutraSweet following a complaint of dumping against its competitor Holland Sweetener, which represented 22% of the European market. The chosen pair received a land-use bonus. Initially, the production of the Gravelines plant was intended for the European market, where large consumers of E951 reside, such as BSN, Pernod-Ricard, Cadbury-Schweppes, Orangina and Coca-Cola. The article added a further detail: "Ajinomoto is not unknown in France, where the group has been associated since 1974 with Orsan (a subsidiary of Lafarge-Coppé) for the manufacture of amino acids." Curious, this marriage between concrete and sweeteners. Not so much, since this group also manufactures industrial glues and therefore solvents.

Before discovering Gravelines, the aspartame *made in France* for Europe, it is necessary to understand that all manufacturers of sodas, food or pharmaceutical products, see the world population increasing to their advantage. With a decrease in the purchasing power of consumers, they are sure to see more and more people eating and drinking for "cheap", before becoming addicted. If the poor "siphoners" of *low-cost* chemistry get sick, they will consume drugs for that purpose and unknowingly taste the good old aspartame again.

The factory that manufactured it for Europe was located in Gravelines, a stone's throw from BASF, the world's leading chemical manufacturer of herbicides, and not far from a nuclear power plant. *Escherichia coli* began producing aspartame for millions of consumers. This created over 100 jobs. Were the aspartame workers informed about the risks of aspartame dust or residues? On the Chinese website Qingdao Twell Sansino Import & Export Co. there is a warning. If the product has a shelf life of two years, it is necessary to "avoid the formation of dust, to keep it away from sources of heat and humidity, and to control the sources of ignition". In Canada, aspartame dust is considered to cause skin, eye and respiratory tract irritation[59] . Just a little history: NutraSweet and Kelco were

---

59. Canadian industry MSDS, First Aid section: "If breathing is difficult, remove victim to fresh air. Give artificial respiration ONLY if the person is not breathing. Give CPR if there is both respiratory arrest and no pulse. Seek URGENT medical attention." Further on, at eye contact: "Do not attempt to give anything by mouth to an unconscious person. If the victim is conscious and not convulsing, rinse the mouth and give one-half to one glass of water to dilute the material..."

married for better or worse, and a December 28, 1999 article in the *Packaging Network* tells us that NutraSweet Kelco's Augusta GA was making aspartame and that during packaging the dust caused some strange environmental pollution. We know nothing more about this aspartame dust affair and little more about the staff of Gravelines who went on strike in 2011 for salary issues and not for possible risks of occupational diseases related to aspartame. However, according to the law of October 25, 1919, a disease can be recognized as an occupational disease if it appears on one of the tables annexed to the Social Security Code. The manufacture of E951 does not appear in the list. Yet in an article in *La Voix du Nord* in November 2014, we learn that an accident occurred in Gravelines, but the investigation was internal and the press was not very talkative: "A subcontractor was doing welding work near a tank containing a substance necessary for the production of aspartame and hydrochloric acid when the incident occurred. The blast from the dry explosion, with no flames, threw the subcontractor to the ground. He was transported conscious and without apparent injury to the CHD."

On Ajinomoto's Euro-Aspartame, we could read: "Respectful of the environment, the company has been ISO 14001 certified since January 2006. In addition, an internal operation plan exists in case of incident or accident (fire, explosion, chemical leakage, injuries...), and exercises are regularly carried out every year."

The expression "dry explosion" may refer to flammable dusts.
No information worthy of the name appeared on the notice board at Gravelines during my visit. The workers were in an informative no-man's land. Doesn't aspartame, especially if it is produced, deserve to be questioned about safety? How many grams of dust can those who make it breathe? Do they wear masks? In Gravelines, the Ajinomoto Sweeteners Europe company located in the Leurette industrial zone has declared to the competent authorities: "The hazard study has shown that the aspartame manufacturing unit does not generate any risk that could have an impact on safety or the environment outside the site: discharges into the atmosphere are limited (use of natural gas as energy, filtration of dust flows, recovery of vapors from the washing and incineration tanks).

Such are the sidelines of the manufacture of aspartame. Next to Ajinomoto's "Eat well, live well", we learn that there was a death in 2011 in the fermenter, but that drills in case of danger were carried out seriously. So no one was in danger of drinking overly aspartame water because "the wastewater is treated in a biological treatment plant, installed on site." Ajinomoto Gravelines received authorization for sludge spreading from the French government in 2009. And users of the compacted sludge were asked to use it only in good weather, i.e. when it is not raining. Ajinomoto was allowed to store its sludge indefinitely and to store it on plots for a maximum of nine or ten months, according to official records. Ajinomoto was tied to each operator, who agreed that his sludge would be "analytically monitored" and subject to unannounced checks. At no time are the words "sweetener manufacturing residues" written. But no farmer has agreed to officially spread the sludge in question on plots located more than 100 km away, where it has mysteriously disappeared... We met the farmers whose plots were notified. They seemed surprised or said they had refused Ajinomoto's offer. If I had not been there, the cadastral plans would have led me to believe that there were existing and very dangerous spreading areas.

The agreement was signed in early 2011:

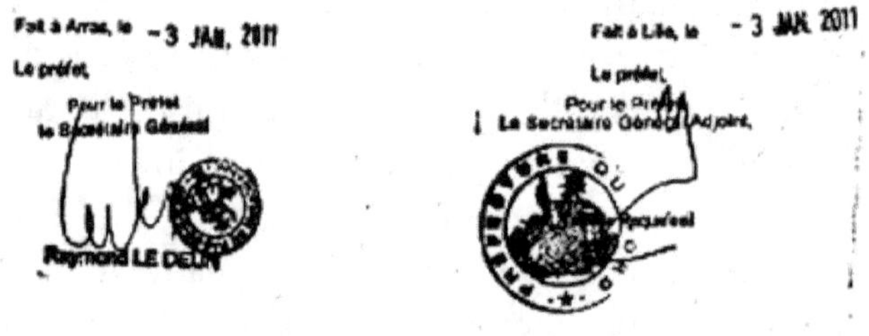

But where is the sludge garbage can located? Has the impact of Ajinomoto on the neighborhood been taken into account to move the sludge far away from its storage? And why is it not where it should be according to the Technological Risk Prevention Plan

(PPRT)[60]. But what does the Japanese group Ajinomoto, which is established throughout the world, really produce? And why does this Japanese giant, associated with Senomyx to test the[61] sugar receptors in humans, now want to leave France and Europe? Because of the laws or because we would not consume enough aspartame anymore? The lawyer of the workers during the eventual closure of the factory, Me Philippe Brun, despite our numerous phone calls, did not deign to answer our questions.

Let us now compare Ajinomoto's aspartame production with the "observant" industry, which respects safety laws. The example of the company Fagron, located in Saint-Denis, in the suburbs of Paris, is exemplary because it is very conscious of the dangers that its employees may face because of aspartame dust and the presence of water. Fagron, a Rotterdam-based company, is a world leader in pharmaceutical preparations; unlike others, its safety data sheet on aspartame is eloquent: aspartame dust can explode and it is its decomposition that is dangerous as well as its contact with water.

SAFETY DATA SHEET
Product : ASPARTAM
COMPOSITION/INFORMATION ON INGREDIENTS
Synonyms: alpha-L-aspartyl-L-phenylalanine methylester, E951
CAS number: 22839-47-0
EC number: 245-261-3
Molar mass: 294.3 g/mol
Gross formula: C14H18N2O5
HAZARD IDENTIFICATION
MAJOR HAZARDS

---

60. The risk prevention plan defined by law n° 2003-699 of July 30, 2003 relating to the prevention of technological and natural risks and the repair of damage is drawn up and adopted by the State, under the authority of the prefect of the department.

61. Before being able to excite the taste buds, the substances must imperatively dissolve in the saliva because the taste receptors only function in a liquid medium. The taste receptors are particularly sensitive chemoreceptors. The sensory information then leaves the taste buds and travels to the brain via the sensory neurons. Researchers have discovered new families of taste receptors. Ajinomoto and Senomyx are working on these genes for Nestlé and other groups and are filing numerous patents.

Not considered as dangerous according to Directive 67/548/EC.
FIRST AID
INHALATION
Get some fresh air.
CONTACT WITH THE SKIN
Wash thoroughly with water. Remove contaminated clothing.
CONTACT WITH THE EYES
Rinse thoroughly with water for at least 15 minutes, holding eyelids apart.
FIRE FIGHTING MEASURES
SPECIFIC RISKS
Possible danger of dust explosion.
MEASURES TO BE TAKEN IN CASE OF ACCIDENTAL DISPERSION
PRECAUTION OF PEOPLE
Avoid dust formation.
ENVIRONMENTAL PROTECTION
Do not discharge to sewer.
CLEANING METHODS
Recover in dry state. Send for disposal
Clean up.
HANDLING AND STORAGE
STORAGE closed, in a dry place.
EXPOSURE/PERSONAL PROTECTION
PERSONAL PROTECTIVE EQUIPMENT
For normal handling, no protection is required.
In case of prolonged exposure to dust, a dust mask is recommended.
Safety glasses can protect against dust.
Wearing gloves is recommended in case of abusive exposure.
STABILITY AND REACTIVITY
DECOMPOSITION PRODUCTS
DANGEROUS
CO_2, CO, NO[62]
TOXICOLOGICAL INFORMATION
Acute toxicity

---

62. An air pollutant once oxidized: nitric oxide.

LD50 (oral, rat): > 5000 mg/kg

In short, we understand that aspartame must remain dry. But where is the sludge from Gravelines being sent? In a region subject to flooding! There is something "wrong" with the reasoning. Having received authorization to spread its sludge on land dedicated to agriculture, except on rainy days, the Ajinomoto company nevertheless received authorization to spread the aspartame and neotame slag in a so-called vulnerable and floodable area! As early as 2009, the prefect of the Nord-Pas-de-Calais region had given his approval for dozens of municipalities for plots far from the production site. The plan was for 6,450 tons of liming and 7,200 tons of composting. This made a total of 13 850 tons. Gone...

I visited Gravelines in early February 2015. The factory that was to be closed in 2014 for relocation to Asia was in full operation. Impossible to meet the new boss who left me the phone number of the switchboard where I was to call him back later. I wanted to know what happened to the sludge that came out of the huge tanks, when it left this valiantly guarded place. In the public inquiry, Ajinomoto had to define its activity to the competent authorities and said:

"SAS Ajinomoto Sweeteners Europe is specialized in the manufacture of aspartame, the aspartame molecule is the result of a reaction between two amino acids: phenylalanine and aspartic acid. The investigation file clearly underlines that the effluents generated are essentially organic aqueous substances and specifies that the products are biodegradable and non dangerous.

But where was the non-hazardous sludge? None of the farmers in the area around Dimont, and this in a vast radius, accepted it. The owners of the plots had often never heard of Ajinomoto's sludge, but of some trucks from the industrial zone of Gravelines, which passed through the area.

Mrs. Chabannes, mayor of Douriez, had come to Gravelines to speak for many mayors of the communes concerned and to express her regret that no meeting had taken place in Pas-de-Calais with the population directly interested in this problem. She was accompanied by the president of a fishing society. After three public posting campaigns, according to the report of the commissaire-enquêteur of April 2, 2009, five communes refused the spreading.

The fishing company Entente de l'Authie was the most virulent in its refusal. The other communes refused the spreading for insufficient guarantees as for the evolution of the decomposition of the sludge. The opinion was unfavorable in Maintenay because of water runoff and groundwater that could be affected. Questions were raised because of the distance and the absence of traceability of the sludge transport. Air pollution was mentioned. In fact, all the municipalities refused the sludge! We can follow those of McCain and Bonduelle, but not those of Ajinomoto. The public investigator had requested an appointment at the Ajinomoto plant. He met with Mr. Hugues Denby Wiljes and the plant manager at the time, Jean-Philippe Loy. He submitted a detailed questionnaire (28 questions), inviting them to respond in writing within twelve days. The following is a summary of the investigation by Mr. Michel Gilmet, who went to the site:

- Why spread so far?
- To avoid mixing too many organic materials in the same area.
- Why did the public inquiry take place in Gravelines and not in the area chosen for the spreading[63] ?
- Municipal councils are free to receive feedback from their constituents.
- Why was the survey sent to the Pas-de-Calais prefecture?
- This is an official deposit.
- Why didn't you hold public meetings?
- They are mandatory if requested...
- Why apply after harvest, when there is no rainfall?
- To protect the water table.
- What are the long-term impacts on soil and crops?
- An agronomic follow-up was requested, in particular a follow-up on the metal content (it is still not known what the Ajinomoto sludge really contains) and a measurement of the residues in winter.
- What is the impact on wildlife?

---

63. The question is really explicit and means: why spread where nobody is consulted!

- Buried sludge limiting contact with wildlife. Sludge is solid, no runoff is expected...

- What is the impact on the flora? The immediate environment, the population and the health risks?

- The composting treatment allows a "hygienization" of the sludge as well as a stabilization in time.

Through the other questions on foul odors, the hydrological study, pollution by runoff, storage points, monitoring, laboratories in charge, we get to the point. We don't know the service provider, but it must be COFRAC accredited and approved by the Water Agency. We don't know why the sludge is not burned in a closed circuit and how the sludge can be used for agricultural purposes. The traceability depends on the SATEGE 62 that we contacted, but which referred us to Ajinomoto. Often the story of aspartame goes in circles, but I persevered. A GIS-type software is provided to track the spills, but it is impossible to locate where the Ajinomoto sludge landed. At the Ramonière landfill near Dimont, some local residents were bothered by the smell. But who knows the smell of a sludge after making aspartame? Has the reclamation of the ecological heritage and the development of agriculture been achieved? How to know? On March 31, 2010, the investigating commissioner Michel Gilmet gave his personal opinion "in his soul and conscience": his report must be taken into account and the code of good practice observed. He issued a favorable opinion to Ajinomoto's request, subject to conditions. But where are the application books? And subject to what control?

The mystery remains about the sludge of sweeteners manufactured on our soil. On June 17, 2015, the hot potato was over: the Dutch company Hyet Sweet[64] bought the plant to produce a new sweetener... The Gravelines site will be named Ajinomoto-Hyet. Hyet Sweet is listed in Gravelines as specializing in the manufacture

---

64. Founded in 2009, this Dutch company, based in Breda, has only five employees. And, unlike Ajinomoto Gravelines, it does not produce but distributes aspartame throughout Europe, and to Coca-Cola and Pepsi. Aelios is financing and supporting the installation of the site.

of basic pharmaceutical products. Hyet is a well-known supplier in the Netherlands. The holding company manufactures erythritol. Discovered in 1874, E968 is a natural sweetener of tetrahydroxy-butane or sugar alcohol. A breath of hope? Will the masters of chemistry finally be concerned about the impact of their productions? Dr. Mercola suggests that too much erythritol can cause severe diarrhea and stomach cramps. If that's all it is...

With no epidemiological studies underway on the effect of aspartame, advantame and neotame, and no specific warnings to physicians, it is time to address the health section.

HEALTH

1 - Research and suspicions

The guarantors of our health claim that the risks are zero. The French advertisement of the Aspartame Information Center uses the usual arguments of harmlessness and the following text is unedited. It is up to you to judge or at least to gauge.

"Myths
"The overwhelming body of scientific evidence clearly demonstrates that aspartame, even in amounts several times higher than what people typically consume, is safe and not associated with adverse health effects. However, over the years, consumers have reported symptoms that they thought were associated with aspartame.

"The FDA investigated these claims and concluded that there was 'no reasonable evidence of possible adverse public health effects' and 'no consistent or unique pattern of symptoms reported in connection with aspartame that may be causally related to its use.

"In 1984, the Centers for Disease Control (CDC) analyzed 517 of these anecdotal reports and stated that "the majority of frequently reported symptoms were mild and were common symptoms in the general population" and that "focused" clinical studies would be the best way to evaluate these complaints.

"As a result, numerous "focused" scientific studies on these claims have been conducted by expert researchers at major academic institutions. The results of these studies have overwhelmingly demonstrated that aspartame is not associated with adverse health effects, including headaches, seizures, mood swings, cognition or behavioral or allergic reactions.

"Despite the overwhelming literature on the safety of aspartame, unsubstantiated claims that aspartame is associated with a myriad of ailments, including multiple sclerosis, Parkinson's disease, Alzheimer's disease, and lupus, have continued to be spread on the Internet and in the media by a few people who have no documented scientific or medical expertise.

"Recently, several governments and expert scientific committees have carefully evaluated the claims posted on the Internet and found them to be false, further reinforcing the safety of aspartame. In addition, leading health authorities, such as the Multiple Sclerosis Foundation, the National Multiple Sclerosis Society, the National Parkinson's Disease Foundation, the Alzheimer's Disease Association and the Lupus Foundation of America have reviewed the Internet claims and have also concluded that they are false."

It can be seen that this statement affirms and clears aspartame of any human pathology other than anecdotal. Consumers can shop with their eyes closed. The story we are being sold is: "Trust us, our researchers are doing the best for your health, we are not hiding anything from you. The FDA has been telling you this since the 1970s..." However, aspartame can be implicated in certain disorders and the list of diseases that some of the medical world attributes to its degradation is not known by doctors who are neither chemists nor toxicologists. Pharmacists would be the best people to help you... But do you have to be an FDA or EFSA expert to have the "real" truth?

List of suspicions:
- Stroke
- Tinnitus
- Allergies
- Alopecia
- Alzheimer's disease
- Anorexia
- Autism
- Bloating (like all sweeteners)
- Logic drop
- Decrease in serotonin

- Sickening need for hydrocarbon (sweet) products
- Cataract
- Cancers
- Blindness
- Coma
- Confusions
- Convulsions
- Cramps
- Crohn's
- Dementia
- Depression (And if the person is on antidepressants, aspartame interacts with them and makes the depression worse).
- Type 2 diabetes and diabetic complications
- Diarrhea
- Joint pain
- Numbness in the legs
- Epilepsy
- Epstein-Barr
- Skin rashes
- Chronic fatigue
- Fibromyalgia
- Excessive hunger and thirst
- Glaucoma
- Retinal gliomas (mothers who abused aspartame)
- Local swelling
- Hyperactivity (children)
- Hyper and hypoglycemia
- Pulmonary hypertension
- Hypothyroidism
- Insomnia
- Burning tongue
- Brain injuries
- Leukemia
- Systemic lupus
- Lyme
- Non-Hodgkin's lymphoma
- Meniere's disease

- Discomfort
- Fetal malformations
- Lack of concentration
- Headaches and migraines
- Myeloma
- Nausea
- Obesity
- Heart palpitations
- Parkinson
- Loss of memory, taste
- Preeclampsia
- Progressive weight gain
- Heart problems (Energy and diet drinks)
- Skin reactions
- Mental retardation (mother ingested aspartame)
- Difficulty breathing
- Retinopathy
- Aneurysm rupture
- Multiple sclerosis (methanol intoxication)
- ALS (Amyotrophic lateral sclerosis, also known as Charcot's disease)
- Unquenched thirst
- Spasms
- Chronic fatigue syndrome
- Post Polio Syndrome
- ADHD or Attention Deficit and Hyperactivity Disorder. It is estimated that 5% of children and 3% of adolescents in France suffer from this disorder.
- Bipolar disorder in adults and children
- Speech problems
- Mood disorders
- Psychic disorders
- Tumors (brain)
- Ulcer
- Dizziness

It is not a question of blaming E951, E950 or E952 for all the evils of the earth, but it can be said that aspartame is a promoter of diseases and that it is involved in certain harmful mixtures. Many people at risk should absolutely avoid taking it.

Aspartame is bad for :
- diabetics (contrary to popular belief),
- obese or overweight people,
- epileptics,
- those who absolutely must not absorb phenylalanine,
- People who have never taken medication and are not aware of their allergy to the product,
- pregnant women,
- children,
- infants,
- fetuses.

But can we know in advance that we are likely to suffer from disorders related to the breakdown of aspartame? The effects and symptoms caused by the leading sweetener have been studied in the laboratory on animals that do not react like humans. The animal would be more tolerant[65] while millions of children around the world become addicted to aspartame. The by-products of aspartame are addictive with an intense withdrawal phenomenon for heavy users of aspartame, when they try to stop consuming it abruptly. Aspartame causes an addiction, and the addiction induces a risk in the more or less long term. In 2003, Dr. Mark Gold of Cambridge sent his report after twenty-five years of studies on the neurotoxic role of aspartame to the FDA. According to him, it caused worrying symptoms ranging from memory loss to brain tumors. But the FDA approval still placed the sweetener in the safe food additive category. Who is to be trusted when the international chemical safety organization INCHEM finds its evaluations and references in Ajinomoto for sweeteners, and Monsanto for pesticides? Yet NutraSweet has

---

65. The fetuses of rats that have ingested aspartame are much smaller and their pancreas does not function normally.

been attacked relentlessly. The excerpt from an article dated August 20, 2005 is worth reading in its entirety[66], as it traces a *class action*, a group of complaints against NutraSweet and Monsanto. The group of plaintiffs sought $350 million. The charges centered on proven racketeering, rigged competition, false advertising, fraud, profanity, and breach of contract on merchandising and warranties. This is what the aspartame industry and consumer confidence is all about...

Amyotrophic lateral sclerosis (ALS) or Charcot's disease is sometimes attributed to aspartame. This sclerosing disease of the nervous system could be caused by methanol which is a neurotoxic. According to doctors, during this disease, motor neurons degenerate, die, cramps appear, muscles lose their volume, language, swallowing and walking are increasingly difficult for the patient. But common symptoms do not necessarily have common causes. Thus, untangling the web of causes is like a *cold case* investigation.

As for E621 and E951, they form a cocktail to which are added pesticides, nitrates, and sometimes strong alcohol. Who can explain the result on our life expectancy? We know that glutamate is a hormonal deregulator of hunger that pushes to eat sweet and promotes obesity, obesity that pushes to consume light: a real vicious circle. And why does aspartame make you hungry? It is because many sweeteners block leptin, the satiety hormone. Leptin is in fact a digestive hormone that regulates our fat reserves, it acts in correlation with another hormone secreted by the duodenum. It acts on serotonin. On the other hand, having a low blood level of leptin statistically predisposes four times more to the risk of Alzheimer's

---

66. *This morning, September 15th 2004, in San Francisco, a $350 million dollar plus class action lawsuit was filed in United States Federal District Court, court case # C 04 3872, against the NutraSweet Corporation, Monsanto Corporation, American Diabetes Association, Dr. Robert H. Moser and some fifty other defendants to be named later. Secretary of Defense Donald Rumsfeld is mentioned throughout in the lawsuit. Rumsfeld was once the CEO and President of G.D. Searle Company which got aspartame approved by the FDA in the 1982. Before taking the CEO position at G.D. Searle, Rumsfeld was Chief of Staff for President Gerald Ford. The question is, did Rumsfeld use his Washington connections to get FDA approval for aspartame when it should not have been approved? [...] The lawsuit contains the following counts : 1. R.I.C.O. (racketeering charges)2. Unfair Competition3. False Advertising4. Consumer Remedies Act5. Fraud6. Breach of Warranty7. Breach of Merchantability8. Filed as a Class Action representing the People as a whole and Joe Bellons personal injuries as well.*

disease. Yet the American Diabetes Association (ADA) recommends aspartame. The diabetologist H. J. Roberts[67], considered that E951 given to diabetics, was equivalent to "delivering salt to the thirsty!" A long policy of burying one's head in the sand has only amplified the promotion of type 2 diabetes and neurological diseases. However, if disorders and diseases occur and are due to sweeteners, neither doctors nor their patients are warned of the risks and interactions with other products. The complexion of the origin of the disorders comes from the fact that an effect can be attributed to one product and its metabolism or to multiple mixtures that are early triggers of a long-term disease. How do we determine the true cumulative culprits? "Let your food be your only medicine, let your medicine be your only food," said Hippocrates."

As a precaution, no one should abuse sweeteners in place of sugar and make the pancreas work in vain. However, during twenty-four hours of a consumer's life, there is a possibility to ingest a lot of sweeteners without knowing it. The prevention of neurological, cerebral or diabetes-related diseases is therefore personal. Regularly absorbed, aspartame plays a role in type 2 diabetes. This has just been partially demonstrated on mice. In the journal *Nature,* it is reported that at the Weizmann Institute in Rehovot, Israel, mice that drink water with sweetener begin to develop glucose intolerance within a few weeks. Sugar substitutes that are supposed to prevent weight gain by limiting the amount of calories absorbed would contribute to the development of metabolic disorders. Researchers at the Weizmann Institute first subjected mice to a diet enriched with sweeteners, successively aspartame, sucralose and saccharin. After eleven weeks, these rodents suffered from hyperglycemia, which was not the case for other mice subjected to a diet without sweeteners. Hyperglycemia is considered one of the early signs of type 2 diabetes, with the development of insensitivity to insulin, a hormone involved in the regulation of the body's energy intake. Consumption of sweeteners by mice disrupts their gut microbes and causes an increase in their blood sugar levels. Suspecting that gut

---

67. Dr. Roberts is a member of the ADA, but he has not been heard despite his obvious conclusions.

bacteria play a role in this effect, the researchers then administered antibiotics to the mice consuming sweeteners, which destroyed their gut flora (or microbiota). To confirm the role of the microbiota in raising blood sugar, the scientists transferred gut bacteria from mice fed a sweetener-enriched diet to mice without microbiota. Six days after the transfer, the recipient mice also suffered from hyperglycemia! The Israeli researchers then studied the reactions of a group of 381 people who were participating in a nutritional study. Those who regularly consumed sweeteners showed various alterations in their metabolism, including hyperglycemia. Finally, they asked seven people who did not normally consume sweeteners to take a week's worth of the usual recommended doses. Four of the participants saw their blood sugar levels rise in just a few days. "It seems that sweeteners have an effect on the body even in the short term," said Dr. Eran Elinav, one of the researchers. As for Luc Tappy, he believes that the number of people who took part in the experiment is too small to draw any conclusion. In any case, it is a first step towards the understanding of the holistic body, of the link between the intestinal flora, the brain, food chemistry and metabolism. Our second brain would be our intestines with neurons[68]. This would explain that brain and intestines can suffer together, from the intestine to the brain, and from the brain to the intestine which has as many neurons as the spinal cord. It is the enteric nervous system that is affected by sweeteners. Michel Neunlist, director of INSERM Unit 913, states that: *"Intestinal neurons are derived from the same embryonic neural plate as the cerebral neurons that form the neural tube and the head. But they colonize the digestive tract from top to bottom, until seven weeks of pregnancy. They then connect to form the networks, without any other structure, just like the encephalon.* One hundred million neurons in the digestive tract, and the enteric network NES is involved."

Scientists in Baltimore have just demonstrated that the gut microbial flora can influence the development of autoimmune diseases such as multiple sclerosis.

---

68. *Science et Avenir*, June 2012. The gut has been dubbed the "second brain" by Michael Gershon, a professor in the Department of Anatomy and Cell Biology at Columbia University in New York.

We now know that the transformation of aspartame in our body can affect the brain, the pancreas, the intestines. Acesulfame-K and sucralose attack the thymus. Sucrose, sucrose and sucralose do not have the same route as sugar. Sugar is recognized by the body's enzymes. Sucralose is absorbed into the bloodstream and almost all of it is found in the urine or feces. 3.3% to 7.2% of sucralose remains in the body after five days. There would be a potential toxicity and risk to our DNA... Sucralose would accumulate in the liver and kidneys. According to Dr. Mercola, the manufacturers of sucralose "don't care about us". Are health insurers and nutritionists lazy or misinformed?

Saccharin can cause bladder cancer and aspartame metabolites are neurotoxic. But there are "chameleon" diseases that can be reactivated by aspartame. Take sexually transmitted Lyme disease. James Bowen explained in 2002 that the immune system gets "lost" with what he calls the twins (Lyme and aspartame). The two together cause autoimmunity, like when the thymus goes haywire with sucralose. A 61-year-old patient had all the symptoms of methyl alcohol poisoning and suffered from horrible allergies. The test for Lyme disease was initially negative, but his bones and cartilage began to break down. The disease (untreated) was sneaking in. All his life, the patient had consumed a diet full of aspartame and the sweetener had caused an immunological disorder and a chemical hypersensitivity syndrome. Both Lyme and aspartame have a "blocking" aspect and distort immune responses. The investigation is progressing slowly, but the extent of misunderstanding is increasing. No one dares to say that some sweeteners are time-delayed poisons. This repeatedly invasive chemistry is not known to the medical profession. According to Dr. Woodrow Monte, author of *While Science Sleeps: A Sweetener Kills*, the death rate increases with aspartame consumption.

Target organ	Formaldehyde target	Affection	Variation over 35 years
Brain	Vascular tissues, Tau protein	Alzheimer's disease	+10 000 %
	Basic myelin proteins	Multiple sclerosis	+100 %
	Vascular tissues, endothelium	Headaches, convulsions	+ ?

	Vascular tissues, endothelium	Glioblastoma tumor	+200 %
Eyes	Retina	Macular degeneration	+30-40 %
Blood vessels	Intima and media of the aorta	Atherosclerosis	+ ?
Skin	Fibroblasts	Skin cancer	+400 %
	Fibroblasts	Dermatitis	+ ?
	Perivascular cells	Lupus	+300 %
Breasts	Epithelium	Adenocarcinoma	+50 %
Kidneys	Epithelium of the tubules	Kidney cancer	+200 %
	Epithelium	Renal overactivity	+100 %
Bones	Synovial membrane	Rheumatoid arthritis	+ after decline
Pancreas	Islets of Langerhans, insulin production	Type 2 diabetes	+1 000 %
Lungs	Fibroblast	Chronic lung disease	+100 %
	Fibroblast	Adenocarcinoma	+ ?
Fetus	DNA methylation	Autism or malformations	+2 500 %
	Liver, lungs, kidneys	Premature delivery	+ ?
Liver	Several targets	Liver cancer	+300 %

Source: Dr. Woodrow Monte

Dr. Monte's graphs leave one wondering: the mortality curves follow one another, and in lightning rises, with a nine-year gap for multiple sclerosis (1990), Alzheimer's starts in 1981, lupus starts in 1979. Brain cancers multiply before the appearance of cell phones in that same year. The autism curve follows that of the consumption of aspartame and starts in 1985, the lesions of the neuronal tube in children, around 1987, the cancers of the kidneys since 1979, of the liver and the lungs in 1980. Cautious, confident or distrustful? The choice is yours.

2 - PROVEN ADVERSE EFFECTS AND NEW LEADS

In the United States, the authorities were obliged to say officially that aspartame was "dangerous for subjects suffering from phenylketonuria", but only in 2003... Depending on the physiological state of an individual, a chemical reaction may not have the same meaning, but how much have the insurances already paid for the damage caused by phenylalanine for example? In high concentrations it acts as a teratogen and the child of a phenylketonuric mother whose diet is not strictly controlled has a very high risk of mental retardation, microcephaly, intrauterine growth retardation and heart malformation and finally premature death. Children suffering from this disease should absolutely avoid aspartame, as the accumulation of the toxic compound damages their brain. How can you follow a strict diet when you don't know what you're ingesting or the effects of the excipients? One of the findings regarding phenylalanine is alarming. Data from animal and human studies suggest a possible chronic effect of high doses of phenylalanine on embryo-fetal development characterized by intrauterine developmental delay, cardiac and visceral malformations and neurological effects[69]. There is more evidence in humans than in animals. According to Dr. Woodrow Monte, the major problem is methanol, which can contribute to chronic diseases. He points out that it has been known since 1940 that methanol is not synthesized in the

---

69. In medical language, it is said that when phenylalanine hydroxylase is absent or strictly reduced, phenylalanine accumulates in the blood and tissues, so that a level of 1000-1200 µmol/l can be reached. The normal level of phenylalanine is 40-120 µmol/l plasma. In children the brain barrier is permeable.

same way by laboratory animals as by humans, and that it is easily transformed into formaldehyde. According to him, some organs are more affected than others.

Pregnant women should not consume aspartame, although E951 is more dangerous for men than for women. In industry, formaldehyde solution is a highly corrosive combustible liquid that must be handled according to the flammable and combustible liquids code. This same formaldehyde crosses the placenta and can be found in breast milk. It is eliminated through the respiratory and renal systems. It is transformed into formic acid, which settles on certain organs such as the kidneys or the brain. But who can really attribute certain diseases or malformations to sweeteners, in particular aspartame? Nobody... So, let's go back to the data acquired from its three main components. Formerly called carbinol or wood spirit, because obtained by dry distillation of wood, methyl alcohol, today called methanol, is a colorless liquid of pleasant odor, miscible with water and acetone. It is used in many chemical syntheses. Methyl alcohol has many uses, including the production of cholesterol, vitamins, hormones and many pharmaceutical products. It is also used as an ingredient in antifreeze for purging brake systems and as an alcohol denaturant, and it is also a dehydrating agent in natural gas. But what could be the link with neurological damage? Until 1981, no influence was visible. The curve of neuronal deficiencies discovered in foetuses followed as if in parallel the consumption of light products, in particular drinks. The two increases coincided perfectly. But the cause could be of any other nature: pollution, heredity, stress, alcohol, drugs, etc., the strongest cause of the deficiencies being fetal alcoholization (but methanol is methyl alcohol.) The peaks of consumption in the United States of the sweetened drinks called *low carb* are precisely in 1994, 1996 and 2000. Did they correspond to an increase in brain deficiencies that can lead to a deterioration of intellectual functioning?

Let's now take the European example. In 1996, in countries like France, there were 721 cases of neuronal deficiencies per 100,000, which gives a total of a little more than 7 cases per 1,000, or 0.07% of babies. Today we are already at more than 1%, and that in less than ten years! Alcohol is likely to cause birth defects or to disrupt development. Today, the average consumption of alcohol per day is 27 g per person in France, compared to 65 g around 1930, and yet cases of neuronal deficiencies are increasing. It is true that women drink more than in 1930, but this does not explain everything. In France, mental retardation is nowadays not only due to alcoholism or lead, so why don't we think about something else, such as aspartame?

The most common mental disorders currently prevalent in many countries are depression, bipolar disorder, schizophrenia and obsessive compulsive disorder. The pattern of consumption often reflects the fact that patients are often lacking many nutrients, essential vitamins, minerals and omega-3 fatty acids. Methanol from aspartame is likely an aggravating factor. What does the dictionary of the Academy of Medicine tell us about the definition of methyl alcohol[70] : that it is an adulterated alcohol and that one should drink alcohol to "dissolve" it in order to protect the nerve cells, the optic nerve, from its transformation into formic acid. In the case of methanol poisoning, the measurement of formates in the urine allows the detection of formic acid metabolized in the body. We know formic acid or methanoic acid if we have walked barefoot on ants. Its name comes from the Latin *formica*, "ants". It is a biological tracer. It is very toxic for the nerve cells...

The ANSES in its February 2013 report made to EFSA adds technical points more complex than the dogma of aspartame "natural and risk-free product": the famous methanol would also play on reproduction, direct alteration of DNA and oxidative stress by accumulation of formic acid. When we assimilate the words,

---

70. "Metabolized into formic acid in the body, it [methyl alcohol] is very toxic for nerve cells: the lesions are elective on the brain and the optic nerve. The accidental absorption of denatured ethanol or methylated spirits, the repeated absorption of adulterated spirits or an unprotected professional exposure is generally the source of intoxications. Following or not a state of drunkenness of ethylic appearance, the signs of gravity appear: agitation, mental confusion, headache and especially narrowing of the visual field. Then there is loss of vision and cyanosis with collapse, sometimes fatal. The emergency treatment consists in the absorption of alcoholic beverages because ethanol (whose metabolism leads to acetic acid, physiological metabolite) displaces methanol and protects the nerve cells against the effects of formic acid. Recovery may leave severe brain and visual sequelae. Methanol can give superacute forms with blindness in twenty-four to thirty-six hours and death in two to three days, and acute forms with more or less complete blindness installed in a few days."

their meanings and the repercussions on our health, understanding is gradually achieved.

Aspartic acid and cysteine appear to create hypothalamic damage, especially in young animals, probably because the blood-brain barrier closes more slowly and never completely around structures like the hypothalamus. The result on mice[71] is obesity and severe behavioral changes. And on the human infant and on the adult?

Everyone knows that aspartame lures the brain by pretending to be a sweet product. But what happens if we stop consuming sugar? On adult rats, the absence of glucose has serious effects. Researchers at Cleveland University School of Medicine fed them *low carb* and studied the results. The rats' blood sugar dropped, their livers began to produce acetone, which was found in the brain instead of sugar. The rats fed with aspartame had protein deficiencies and their brains were damaged. This neurological study dates back to 1995. A period of prolonged fasting or diabetes causes ketogenesis. Ketone bodies are formed, including acetylacetic acid, which is involved in lipid metabolism. The imperfect breakdown of fatty acids can lead to ketonemia, or ketonuria. This is usually treated with insulin therapy. In other words, without the right fuel, our body, fooled by internal solvents and overdoses of credulity, does not feel very good.

According to the American study, "Birth defects caused by aspartame", mothers who drank too much *Diet Cola* during their pregnancy could give birth to babies with deformed skulls or hydroce-phalus. These babies, whose skulls can reach 91 cm in circumference, are victims, like laboratory mice... *Low carb* is nonsense, because it takes energy, not formalin and formic acid, for a baby's and mother-to-be's brain. The subject remains complicated, but some data now make it accessible. As a simple journalist, I went to dig up a lot of information to find the substance and stop beating around the bush. We now know that formaldehyde is mutagenic and carcinogenic by combustion, that it promotes bronchial asthma, causes leukemia and respiratory cancers and that it was therefore classified as a definite carcinogen in 2004 by the International Agency for Research on

---

71. Photographs can be found in profusion on the Internet.

Cancer. And that induced by the consumption of aspartame would not be harmful? Diseases would only have symptoms and no causes?

A recently unnoticed industry decision reveals a form of awareness: in 2013, Pepsi-Cola launched its diet drink without aspartame. The manufacturer reversed course in silence, seeming to have gone from minimal distrust to maximum caution by stopping E951 in its diet drinks. Is it the story of the young star who represented Pepsi-Cola light, which convinced the manufacturer to stop using it? This young world-famous actor was affected by Parkinson's disease at a very early age. In a letter addressed to the famous American presenter Oprah Winfrey, Betty Martini exposed the fact that Michael Fox - that's him - suffered from this disease since he had promoted the drink in question. The cause of Michael Fox's illness was probably related to his addiction to Diet Pepsi. Michael Fox was for a long time the spokesman and the muse of *Diet Pepsi* which he had abused by taste and addiction. The hero of *Back to the Future*, then a star who fell from the firmament, was not yet 30 years old when he was struck by an irreparable disease. His image became counterproductive. After having praised Diet Pepsi as a must, he developed Parkinson's disease. In 2000, he founded the Michael J. Fox Foundation for Parkinson's research, the day before the last episode of the series *Spin City was* broadcast. Is he living proof that aspartame is a promoter of early neurological disease? Is this why the new diet drinks, like Next Pepsi, no longer contain a trace of aspartame?

Normally, Parkinson's disease occurs before the age of 60, and it is very unusual before the age of 30, yet less and less rare. A mixture of genetic and environmental causes, the disease is due to a lack of dopamine in the brain. Many academic studies indicate that aspartame lowers dopamine levels. Too much aspartame would cause dopamine and serotonin levels in the brain to drop. Was Michael Fox a victim of this effect? Can Parkinson's disease be triggered by aspartame in an even younger age group? This is the worrying question.

The American food group PepsiCo had announced on April 24, 2015 its official decision to abandon the use of aspartame in the production of its sugar-free and calorie-free drinks. But this only applied to the United States, and consumers were snorting so much they were used to the old drink without worrying about teenagers and children with juvenile Parkinson's syndrome. Cramps, walking disorders and uncontrolled movements are the symptoms of this disease. The point of detail that attracts attention is that the drug Parlodel, first-line treatment for Parkinson's disease[72] and antilactation (Pfizer and Meda Pharma), prohibits the joint intake of aspartame or the intake of the drug Zyprexa (which also contains aspartame), it can cause a coma. Same thing for Celance from Lilly Laboratories, Requip (GSK) and Tasmar (Tolcapone) suspended and put back on the market in 1994. These antiparkinsonian drugs in the presence of aspartame would be excessively dangerous! Parlodel was, until recently, prescribed by gynecologists... No serious literature on the subject of Parkinson and E951 has appeared to me.

In France, an actress adored by the French, was addicted to Diet Coke, and what did she die of? From Alzheimer's disease. Diet Coke was the "drug" of Annie Girardot on the shootings. According to Coca-Cola, a can of diet Coke contains 80 mg of aspartame for 33 cl. According to Devra Davis, there would be up to 200 mg per can.

Another deficiency would be due to aspartame: autism. As early as 1983, it was noticed that the number of autistic people in the United States was increasing and that it followed the consumption of aspartame. Four years later, it exceeded it. If we compare alcoholism and "aspartamism", the symptoms linked to the absorption of aspartame double those of alcohol as early as 1984. A new evaluation in the United States on subjects aged 6 to 17 years showed an increase in autism cases from 0.7 ‰ to 5.3 ‰ from 1996 to 2007. By 2003 the rate was 1 in 450! Today, according to the Pasteur Institute, worldwide, 1 in 100 children is autistic... 1 in 50 in many U.S. states.

On rats, there is talk of damage that can cause autism, but on the packages of diet drinks that children can drink, there is no mention of anything so sad and terrifying. Only on rats... Rats don't go to

---

72. This drug was also authorized to stop lactation after childbirth or to stop it after breast-feeding. Bromocriptine (Parlodel® and Bromocriptine Zentiva®) should no longer be prescribed in this indication, according to a decision published by the French drug agency on July 25, 2013. (See Medisite's website on childbirth-breastfeeding-the-parlodel-c-is-finished.)"

school, so why test on lab rats? Need we remind you that children are meant to live without mental disabilities, not to be guinea pigs for any addiction? And what do we know about the impact of metabolites on the unborn child? Charles Kokoski, now retired, while head of the Food Addictives Evaluation Branch, received a letter from Thomas F. X. Collins about the damage of aspartame on animals, only on animals. Collins had noticed strange abnormalities: "At high doses, the eyes seem to be affected...The fetuses show remarkable changes in the sense of unusual, such as a bony diminution of vertebrae and phalanges and even cases of hydrocephalus."

With an ingestion of 2 g, they suffered severe malformations. Aspartame did not appear to be lethal to rabbits and lab mice at these extreme doses. But this meant that aspartame could cause monsters to be born but did not kill them. To claim that aspartame is teratogenic, you need really "deadly" evidence! On Doctissimo, a general public site, future mothers are worried and wonder. A general practitioner answers them that from the age of 10, it is without risk. Why not before, if it is not dangerous? Because the cranial barrier is still fragile? On this discussion site, we find this testimony: "Working in the field of preventive medicine for more than fifteen years, I can only support the advice to absolutely avoid the consumption of sweeteners of any kind. Aspartame contains, among other things, methanol, which turns into a toxic element at 34°C. Sweeteners cause a cephalic insulin reflex. The pancreas produces insulin when no sugar is really present. As a result, the body craves more and more "sweet" foods. I have observed that people who cut out these sweeteners can lose weight rapidly in a relatively short period of time. In summary: aspartame, which can be found in diet products, toothpastes, ready meals, pickles, mustard but also in livestock feed, makes you fat!!!"

The Canderel website provides answers to a mother's concern: "I am pregnant or breastfeeding: is aspartame dangerous for my health or my baby's?" Canderel reassures, "Aspartame is safe for pregnant women and infants." And further on, the same refrain repeated:

"The link between aspartame and pregnant women has been the subject of several evaluations by numerous health authorities, such as the European Food Safety Authority (EFSA) or the World

Health Organization (WHO): there is no contraindication for pregnant women who wish to consume aspartame, no risk for the fetus. Finally, the consumption of aspartame has no harmful effect on breast milk.

The worldwide addiction to aspartame has taken hold, this "miracle" product may in time turn out to be a global health disaster. The sweetener liner is a silent *Titanic*. Before sinking, it will have made a lot of money for its manufacturers. However, the marketing of aspartame is not a conspiracy, it is even an absence of conspiracy, because its industry has imposed itself over the years. This empire is not afraid of being pushed around by whistleblowers, it has simply informed the medical profession through its "experts" and let citizens do their shopping. The rare recalcitrant ones are considered as agitated. It is so easy to "believe" in the good word of industrialists who already feed more than a billion gullets, they can well lose a few handfuls of refractory who do not make noise... Nothing to worry about since nobody officially says that neuronal degeneration can be linked to aspartame; but if a person supposedly suffering from Alzheimer's regains his memory by stopping taking it, it is the proof that his symptoms did not have a genetic origin! Let's remember that aspartame would cause tumors of the urinary tract, an increase in the rate of brain cancer, metabolic acidosis mimicking diabetic ketoacidosis, liver and lung cancer, a possible increase in cancer gene expression in the organs, negative effects on spatial cognition and insulin sensitivity, etc. And here the investigation progresses between fat and brain! According to a 2011 study conducted by Egyptian researchers involving mice, it can be understood that subcutaneous administration of aspartame, alone or in the presence of mild systemic inflammatory stress, increases oxidative stress and inflammation in the brain. Oxidative stresses are responsible for neurodegenerative diseases. Yet aspartame continues to be given to diabetics in nursing homes, with the blessing of the medical profession.

Is sucralose better? E955, a product recommended for diabetics, is said to attack the thymus[73] and cause it to shrink by 40%, double

---

73. The thymus is a granular gland, a butterfly-shaped "wart", well below the neck. This mysterious lock is extremely important. *Thymos* means "soul" and "spirit" in Greek.

the risk of decline in renal function in women, increased risk of non-Hodgkin's lymphoma and multiple myeloma, enlarged liver and kidneys, reduced growth rate, and to contribute to symptoms of fibromyalgia, abnormal pelvic mineralization, and pelvic hyperplasia Studies on animals have shown that at high doses, sucralose can involve not only a reduction in the size of the thymus but also in the intestinal flora. Other studies show other pathologies: psychotic panic, muscle pain, diarrhea, bloating, intestinal pain, stomach pain and bladder problems. The thymus, a soft organ weighing only a few grams, is the nursery of the immune system; it is there that the T lymphocytes mature. Without this army of micro-soldiers, we would be in constant danger. However, there are autoimmune diseases such as myasthenia, where the lymphocytes produce antibodies against the patient's own acetylcholine receptors. When the receptors are destroyed, the nerve impulses are no longer transmitted and muscle contraction is no longer possible. The causes of the immune system dysfunction in myasthenia remain an enigma. Not all the factors responsible for an autoimmune disease are known, but it is mainly in the thymus that the lymphocytes learn to tolerate the constituents of our body and not reject them as foreign bodies. In the case of autoimmune disease, we speak of a genetic predisposition. This is an argument that sweetener manufacturers use, they can't help it if you have a predisposition to diabetes, autoimmune diseases or allergies... And a disease with multifactorial origins can have genetic factors that combine with environmental factors. In other words, there is a lack of a guide to sweeteners that may promote an underlying disease. But then, they would not be sold anymore. Conflicting information thus paves the way for this investigation, and it is up to the medical profession and its own brains to take it up. To sweeten means to soften, to temper, to remove, to subtract... Aspartame instead of removing a risk, adds some that remain undetectable.

3 - Aspartame, the body, the brain and toxicology

What is going on inside us without our being aware of it? With marvelous precision, every day the body produces a certain amount of energy which is initially contained in fats (lipids), proteins (protids) and sugars (carbohydrates). Food and reserves allow the body to manufacture energy essential to life. These reserves are in the form of glycogen for sugar inside the liver, fatty acids for fats inside the adipose tissue, and proteins inside the muscles. Energy metabolism is a source of calories but also of waste. Urea is an example. These residues are most often acidic. The body constantly expels carbon dioxide, hydrogen and substances from the breakdown of certain cells. A small part of them agglomerates elsewhere before disappearing or not.

Acetone comes from cells that are deficient in sugar. The so-called "buffer system" is there to neutralize the acidifying power of substances carried by the blood within the general circulation system and it would be dangerous for the brain to be soaked in acetone... The term acidosis refers to the impossibility of properly eliminating excess acid. It comes either from a defect of elimination, or from an excess of production, as it is the case for example during diabetes which is complicated by a diabetic coma or ketoacidosis. Terms reserved for the medical profession gradually become audible. Everything fits together logically when we study formulas that we did not know before. Let's take the case of acidosis, it can be the result of intoxication by a drug, even the simplest one like aspirin (acetylsalicylic acid). But is there such a thing as acidosis due to *sweet light* slag in diabetic subjects? Acute metabolic complications sometimes reveal diabetes and there are about 50 cases of diabetic ketoacidosis per 10,000 diabetics in Western countries.

Knowing that methanol is a better solvent than ethanol, and that formic acid results from the ingestion of aspartame, can E951 be freely consumed without restriction by diabetics? Polish doctors J. Szponar, A. Górska, M. Majewska, M. Tchórz, G. Drelich, made a strange discovery that partly answers this question. They saw a man in his sixties arrive in the emergency room with a life-threatening prognosis. The medical staff suspected methanol poisoning because the patient had symptoms of diabetes with extreme hyperglycemia and coma, a coma characterized by massive dehydration. Laboratory tests showed metabolic acidosis[74] and respiratory acidosis and methanol and ethanol levels of 80 mg/dl and 0.47 g/l. Doctors diagnosed excessive consumption of aspartame as the cause of the poisoning. In a further study, they hypothesized that long-term consumption of aspartame could accelerate atherosclerosis and cellular aging.

Another experiment that proves the involvement of aspartame is a study on a family of zebrafish, conducted by Korean scientists to determine the physiological effect of aspartame in the presence of hyperlipidemia in the laboratory, which approximates the condition of overweight or obese people. Zebrafish[75], also known as "pyjamas", were fed either aspartame or saccharin, each sweetener combined with a high cholesterol diet. The results showed that in the presence of hyperlipidemia, fish fed aspartame showed abnormalities in movement with increased brain inflammation. 30% of these fish

---

74. Acidosis which can also be due to fasting, uncontrolled diabetes mellitus.

75. Source: AFP of April 18, 2013, article by Caroline Albert: "Researchers have decoded the genome of the zebrafish, a "model organism" commonly used in laboratories to study human diseases, and discovered that 70% of the genes of the small fish have an equivalent with ours. This genome is the largest ever decoded in a vertebrate (26,000 coding genes). And it has been sequenced with such a degree of precision "that we can really make direct comparisons between human and zebrafish genes," says Derek Stemple, a geneticist at the Wellcome Trust Sanger Institute in Cambridge, UK...." Zebrafish (*Danio rerio*) have long been used as models for studying human diseases, in part because they are easy to raise in large numbers in the laboratory. In addition, their embryos develop outside the mother and are transparent, allowing easy observation of their cellular development.

died prematurely, while all those fed saccharin survived. The aspartame-fed fatty fish had an increase in serum atherogenic lipid profile[76] with an increase in the activity of cholesterol ester transfer proteins. The choice is not between plague and cholera, saccharin or aspartame, but between eating well. To understand the sprawling subject of aspartame, one must find scientific information that at first glance seems unfathomable, but which is very instructive and suddenly simplifies the reasoning.

Everywhere in our body, biochemical exchanges are working or not. Some amino acids are only provided by food, which is why they are called essential amino acids, and phenylalanine is one of them. Others are produced by the organism, it is the case of tyrosine, which is both brought by the food and also manufactured by the organism from phenylalanine. Tyrosine plays a fundamental role in the management of physical and mental activity. Its deficiency causes depression, hyperactivity, sleep disorders and thyroid disorders. Tyrosine is derived from phenylalanine and is a phenol. The transformation of phenylalanine into tyrosine takes place mainly in the liver with the action of enzymes. Phenylketonuria is a genetic disease that is prolonged by a dysfunction of these enzymes. That is why those who suffer from it should not take aspartame, a source of phenylalanine. It is not bad in itself, it is dangerous for some and sometimes fatal.

Tyrosine Kinases are involved in tumor progression. These receptors are now studied by the CNRS Molecular Biology Research Center under the name SRC. Tyrosine is a non-essential amino acid, which takes its name from *Tyros*, "cheese" in Greek, and which has a major role in the nervous system. It controls appetite, stress and blood pressure. If we lack it, we can suffer from emotional disorders, physical or intellectual fatigue, depression, drowsiness, lack of concentration, stress, skin lesions and a decrease in the production of thyroid hormones which control the basic metabolism. An overdose

---

76. Atherogenic is what accelerates the process of degenerative alteration of the internal vessel wall with the formation of a plaque of lipid deposits, and also by the release of lipoid crystals and cholesterol, and then by sclerosis of the affected area that may calcify or ulcerate. Serum proteins are proteins contained in the serum and blood plasma that protect the body, transport and regulate.

causes almost the same thing as a deficiency. Tyrosine from phenyla-lanine can cause an excess of dopamine. Aspartame, apparently, contains a dreaded medicine cabinet. It can have a harmful role for the sight in certain people. Professor H. J. Roberts was convinced that it caused black flashes in front of the eyes, double vision, eye pain, bleeding and tears in the retina, and cataracts. The latter, in their early stages, can be stopped only by stopping the intake of aspartame[77]. According to Professor Roberts, aspartame leads to an acceleration of clinical diabetes and the worsening of diabetes-related complications. "Unfortunately, many of my patients seen in consultation develop serious metabolic, neurological complications that could be specifically attributed to the use of aspartame-containing products," he lamented.

Russell Blaylock stated that the excitotoxins caused by aspartame could accelerate diabetes in subjects genetically susceptible to this disease. Dr. John Olney, a professor of neuropathology and psychiatry in Missouri, had documented clinical cases of aspartame in combination with monosodium glutamate, which increased brain damage in children. Dr. Mercola made the point, but so did an army of researchers[78]. Excitotoxins are slow poisons. In France, we have the list of excipients with notorious effects (EENS), a list updated in 2009 and elaborated by the AFFSAPS (French Agency for Health Products Safety). It contains phenylalanine and aspartame but the official note only mentions the danger for people suffering from phenylketonuria. However, in the child suffering from phenylk-etonuria, the toxicity of phenylalanine is proven only after birth. Professor François Feillet said in 2006: "Untreated, phenylke-tonuria leads to mental retardation sometimes profound as well as depigmentation, a controlled diet in phenylalanine allows patients to lead an almost normal life. Phenylalanine has a developmental toxicity, with the occurrence of severe embryofoetopathy in the children of women with untreated phenylketonuria during their

---

77. For more information: *Sunshine Sentinel Press*, P.O. Box 17799 West Palm Beach, Florida 33416.

78. Kate S. Collison, Nadine J. Makhou, Marya Z. Zaidi, Rana al-Rabiah, Angela Inglis, Bernard L. Andres, Rosario Ubungen, Mohammed Shoukri, and Futwan A. al-Mohanna in their work on nutrition and metabolism at Riyadh Hospital, Saudi Arabia.

pregnancies. These women should be informed and pregnancies should be planned with resumption of the diet in the preconceptional period. Routine neonatal screening has been implemented in the United States because of its incidence (1 in 17,000 cases) and *the* availability of effective treatment. Since 1970, approximately 1600 phenylketonurias have been diagnosed and treated.

On a billion of regular consumers, wouldn't it be a small sanitary risk? The cause of phenylketonuria is partly alimentary. The prevalence of this disease varies from 1 case for 3,000 to 30,000 according to the countries. Recently, it was 1 case for 50,000. This sudden increase is due to an overdose of phenylalanine. The brain constitutes 2% of the body mass of the human body and fears overdoses of sugar and sweeteners; and what is proven in children is that a deficiency due to aspartame seems irreparable. Everyone knows that hypoglycemia creates anxiety, but no one suspects that many hyperactive children actually suffer from a diet full of synthetic sweeteners that contain neither vitamins nor minerals.

Another common sense reminder: fruits are naturally sweet, and this sugar is always accompanied by vitamins (B1) and minerals (magnesium) essential to their metabolization. However, we can be addicted to refined sugar which contains neither minerals nor vitamins. It forces our body to draw these vitamins and minerals from its own reserves (such as the calcium in our bones). Another interesting fact: diabetes probably accelerates brain aging. This is the conclusion of the Aric study (United States), which dates from 1987. Prevention of diabetes limits the number of cases of dementia. But what if diabetes was really promoted by aspartame leading to neurological diseases? Alzheimer's costs 129 billion euros each year in the United States, according to a 2010 estimate. However, with the aging of the population, and according to the same source, this amount should increase by 80% by 2040.

How does fake sugar lure your brain? It starts with a beautiful advertising poster that activates the complexes of each one. The *sweet light*, in candy bars or in drinks, then feigns our natural computer. The brain takes a liking to it. This not very heavy organ is very greedy in glucose which it needs seriously. It consumes 20% of the energy necessary for our basic metabolism, i.e. the energy necessary

3 - Aspartame, the body, the brain and toxicology

for the body to live a day without physical activity. The reserves of our natural computer are only ten minutes. When we exert ourselves, our brain cries out for energy. And when our "captain" is deficient, he causes a decrease in cognitive faculties, which can lead to aberrant behavior. Insulin evolves according to blood sugar peaks and when blood sugar levels rise with meals, insulin secretion increases immediately, allowing sugar to enter the cells. Our brain acts like an automatic pilot for the well-being of our body. Fooled by E951, it is no longer "itself". Lying to the brain is to lead it from error to error, and the one that "monitors and directs" believes it is doing the right thing and gives the order for insulin secretion. This phase is called CPIR, *cephalic-phase insulin release*. It seems to be well demonstrated that when breakfast is not balanced in carbohydrates, there are losses at the cognitive level (memory and vigilance).

People with diabetes need less sugar because their insulin cannot metabolize it. Diabetes is a disease characterized by high levels of glucose or blood sugar in the blood. Being overweight contributes to the link between diabetes and dementia because the fatty tissue that builds up with weight gain reduces the effectiveness of insulin in the body, which can affect the activity and health of brain cells. If ingested aspartame promotes weight gain and is dangerous to the brain, that means diabetics are at risk if they consume it. This is a kind of double punishment for them, because instead of helping them to live better, we make them more fragile. Why does this logic escape its prescribers? It is not only the weight, because since the appearance of the super-aspartame called neotame, brain tumors would have increased in the United States.

Now that we know that aspartame is a lure for the brain, it is interesting to understand the internal process. The neurotransmitters released by the taste buds in the taste neurons, are information transmitted to the brain by three cranial nerves. Our deluded central regulator believes that it is real glucose, but the sweetener does not have the same effects on memory and energy! Our malnourished brain then goes on alert, bluffed, as brilliant as it is, it starts looking for energy. The victim, as soon as he can, will eat sugar, order of his brain regulator ... Two soft drugs therefore that the false sugar and the real refined sugar ...

The chemical exchanges in our body factory as well as the whole of the molecular and energetic transformations which take place in an uninterrupted way in our cells escape us. How many food additives per day or over the years disrupt our metabolism? Biochemists can explain the breakdown of aspartame, but can they assess the consequences of its ingestion? Biochemistry is a very complex science and spectrometry now tells us what your brain has to sort out and how it does. According to two researchers from Compiègne, in vivo magnetic resonance spectrometry of the proton makes it possible to quantify a cellular suffering by the analysis of certain metabolites. Future tools in perspective will undoubtedly offer certain keys, until now ignored. In any case, aspartame having lured the brain all year long, the latter does not cease to compensate, and gorges itself when it can. The "sweetening" acaloric products therefore produce the opposite effect. Two American nutritionist researchers, Professor Terry Davidson and his associate, Professor Susan Swithers, fed two groups of rats for ten days either with sweetened liquids or with sweetened liquids. Both groups of rats could choose what was more tempting for them. After ten days, those who received the sweetener ate more chocolate... Now, diet sodas have been all the rage for a very long time, especially in the United States. In the country of the first *sweet light* products, the number of overweight consumers represents nearly 60% of the population! The theory according to which aspartame allows you to lose weight because of the absence of sugar is now losing its substance. CQFD... The light, it is really heavy, but we still have many things to discover before pronouncing or accusing in conscience. Why do many scientists use the conditional about the responsibility of aspartame in certain diseases? Do they not dare to think for themselves or do they not take the warnings seriously? However, a too long and strong absorption of intense sweeteners can cause Alzheimer's disease, which continues to progress in the world. Lilly laboratories would have found a molecule that would slow down the degeneration process, especially in patients who have not yet developed symptoms. Lilly began its research in the 1990s on memory disorders. "Delaying the onset of the disease by five years would save society $447 billion a year until 2050," said Michael Hutton, scientific director of neurodegenerative diseases at the same laboratory. With other public and private laboratories, Lilly is working on the development of biomarkers, in particular to indicate the probability of the occurrence of the pathology. If aspartame causes the disease for some people, and these Monsanto and now Bayer associates take care of it, we can sleep "peacefully": they are going to attack neurofibrillary degeneration, another feature of the disease, targeting the Tau protein that accumulates abnormally in the neurons. The further we go, the more new areas there are to understand. There are several explanations for the "crazy" behavior of Tau proteins: phosphorylation of this protein which contains little phosphorus but which leads to its accumulation, oxidative stress which alters the neuronal walls by modifying calcium movements, genetic factors and age. Degeneration is caused by the death of millions, then billions of neurons, with loss of memory. It can lead to dementia. Tau proteins are normally found in neurons to stabilize axons. They are also present in the presynaptic terminals. These proteins are very important and are coded by genes located on our chromosomes: their coding obeys complex biochemical and molecular mechanisms in order to assume normal life or death functions of the cells. Together, they lead to what is called "tauopathy". Tauopathies are rare and very challenging and relatively early onset diseases according to Canadian doctor Nathan Herrmann. According to Professor Marie-Pierre Thibodeau and her team, it is "imperative that clinicians understand the molecular neuropathology of these various syndromes. It is about "intraneuronal aggregation of abnormally phosphorylated Tau proteins, a degenerative process that affects the hippocampal region", as pointed out by predictive medicine specialists from Lille, Luc Buée and André Delcourte, back in 2002.

According to the Quebec journalist Sophie Allard, "when the disease strikes in the thirties, the severity of the symptoms progresses at a lightning speed. It would be of genetic origin, but why are there more cases of Alzheimer's[79] today than in the past and especially

---

79. For the record, here are some of the symptoms of Alzheimer's disease: 1) Memory problems; 2) Difficulty with daily tasks; 3) Language problems; 4) Spatial and temporal disorientation; 5) Poor judgment; 6) Difficulty with abstract thinking; 7) Misplaced objects; 8) Mood changes; 9) Personality changes; 10) Loss of initiative.

in countries with a high consumption of new food products that contain thousands of aspartame... The disease is recognizable by the lesions that characterize it, amyloid plaques and neurofibrillary clusters. This disease affects an average of 5% of people under 65, 10% of people over 65, 20% of people over 80, 40% of people over 85. It is a neurodegenerative dementia that primarily affects cognitive functions and has an impact on the behavior and social adaptation of patients. One can imagine the financial abyss and the distress of the families. And for oneself, one fears to be reached by this disease "before the legal age". In France, early-onset Alzheimer's affects 1% to 3% of patients under the age of 60. The disease is characterized by certain factors including hyperphosphorylation of the Tau protein, a reduction in the use of glucose in the brain (probably due to a decrease in insulin receptors), oxidative stress, inflammation, mercury, etc. The neurological and behavioral degradations of the disease are multifactorial. So it is essential to sort out, and above all, multifactorial prevention if aspartame is part of it! Alzheimer's disease has a wide variety of origins, so, as one advertisement said, "no need to add to it". It took millennia for man to refine his immune defenses and his metabolism, and a simple sweetener would have the right to undo everything?

Testimonials

In ancient times, many centenarians died in perfect health, like Pythagoras, and with "all their wits about them". We are increasingly ill and dependent on medication. Body shape and fitness have always been linked to lifestyle and aspartame is a false remedy that is far from certain basic principles. We walk less, eat too fast, and as a Greek proverb says, "Health and reason are the two treasures of mankind." French sayings remind us, "The man with less excess has better health. The poor have health, the rich have remedies." So are the risks associated with aspartame in areas such as obesity, neurology, autism, or life expectancy greater or lesser than the benefits? Not being a doctor or a pharmacist, I wanted to know if stopping aspartame had a positive influence on health. During the writing of this book, I asked several people around me who suffered from several disorders that are attributed to aspartame (glaucoma, fatigue, neurological disorders, depression, etc.) what they drank, and even if it is not worth anything scientifically speaking, I would like to say that two thirds of them drank Diet Coke and were diabetic, and all of them took aspartame daily. One of them had glaucoma, was addicted to aspartame and diet, and her anti-smoking gums contained it; Dominique L. could not stop taking these products. Now, she is no longer addicted to aspartame and has replaced it with stevia. The second one, diabetic, stopped taking aspartame that she used to put everywhere, in her coffees and cakes, and replaced it by tagatose. Three months later, she had lost weight, her speech was better and her standing was better. A year later, she had lost weight again and her speech was much better. She was diagnosed with a degenerative orphan disease. She was losing her balance and having difficulty expressing herself to the point of seeing a speech therapist. "I will never take aspartame again", Sonia B. told me, even though the medical profession had strongly advised her to do so, and she was putting it everywhere. Since Sonia B. stopped taking aspartame, her life has improved. The third person belongs to a family of diabetics, all using aspartame and suffering from depressive episodes. Anne D., a friend who had to go on a diet to preserve her heart and therefore her health, had to stop consuming sugar. The medical specialist advised her to take aspartame. I talked her out of it!

Have pregnant women with diabetes been considered? Knowing a mother-to-be with type 1 diabetes, I noticed that the hospital world did not ban sweeteners. I went on the Internet to see what was said on this subject. On the Doctissimo site, it says, "Despite diabetes, you can be a foodie...and sweeteners can be valuable allies for risk-free taste pleasure." Even for pregnant women with type 1 or 2 diabetes? The mentioned site speaks about absence of risk concerning the glycemia, but does not speak about the rest, of the metabolites crossing the placenta, reaching a baby's brain. The Canadian site Dispensaire diététique de Montréal warns about something else, sweeteners are not dangerous for pregnant women "except for cyclamates and glycyrrhizin". As for glycyrrhizin, it is recognized as GRAS and safe by the FDA while it can harm the development of the child. In short, who cares what a fetus ingests? On the babycenter website, it says that "sweeteners are safe during pregnancy". However, the site recommends not to abuse them to avoid bloating and intestinal gas. But nothing for diabetic mothers, except on a dedicated site, that of the Federation of Diabetics. Becoming a mother when you have diabetes, whatever the type of diabetes, is possible, but it cannot be improvised! "If diabetes and pregnancy can be reconciled, diabetic pregnancy remains a risky pregnancy. With a planned pregnancy, a good glycemic balance from the moment of conception and a specific adapted follow-up, you will put all the chances on your side for you and your child. Further on: "Hypoglycemia and hyperglycemia will inevitably occur during your pregnancy, you should try to avoid them as much as possible and when they do occur, make sure they do not last." So it's advisable to see a diabetologist if you're pregnant. But what if the diabetologists don't know the risks? On the diabetic women's site, it is suggested that "0% fruit yogurt with no added sugar (for acceptance of gestational diabetes and the associated diet, a yogurt with sweetener is suggested for women who can not do without the sweet taste)." This sentence is contradicted further on by a testimony of a mother-to-be: "Goodbye to sweet products: ice cream, pastries, chocolate, cookies, sweetened and even sweetened drinks because sweeteners are not recommended during pregnancy."

The following testimony comes from the mother of a young epileptic who committed suicide. Mrs. Libor lives in the Jura region and she wishes to participate in this investigation with her testimony: "In the early 1980s, we temporarily replaced white sugar with zero-calorie aspartame. Our daughter, 6 or 8 years old at the time, was epileptic, and her treatment (Depakine[80]) made her gain weight. The fake sugar "forced" her to find food all the time. What a mistake! My husband and I were able to observe a decrease in our daughter's vision and hearing. This chemical (which I also used) made my muscle pain worse, I had been suffering from macrophage myofasciitis[81] since early childhood. It's awful how often we are deceived, cheated..."

This is just a testimonial about a drug that makes you fat and pushes you to take aspartame to limit your calorie intake. This person's daughter died. And no one to explain how the vicious circle was established that pushed her to a desperate act. In this letter, one feels the distress born of vagueness and contempt. What is not obvious is the disabling neuromuscular degenerative disease called "myofasciitis". What characterizes it are food intolerances to gluten, lactose, aluminum, and aspartame. Who thinks of the unfortunate people who are intolerant to aspartame? Profitability would suggest not to ask too many questions when tens of thousands of tons of it

---

80. Anti-epileptic when benzodiazepines proved ineffective in preventing seizures, now accused of causing birth defects, its prescription was restricted in late May 2015.

81. Macrophage myofasciitis is a rare disease identified in 1993 by Michelle Coquet. A controversy exists, because the disease is more often associated with the pathological persistence of aluminum salts, but the AFFSSAPS affirmed that there is no link and that it would be an auto-immune disease.

are manufactured every year in the world. The Ugandan ambassador to the World Environment Conference on Aspartame assured Laurie Moser that the Ugandan sugar industry was adding aspartame to sugar and that the son of one of the industry's leaders could not walk, presumably because of his gluttony for E951, which turned into overdosing. He would have eaten it like sugar powder. But this probable poisoner remains available to the world to talk to our taste buds... Other testimonies are more snarky. The Mills family in the United States, Georgia, is convinced that aspartame has wreaked havoc in their midst. The son was born with neurological problems, his mother Karen had been exposed during her pregnancy to excessive doses of NutraSweet, Diet Coke, and Diet 7 Up, as well as pills with phenylalanine, in short, a deleterious cocktail! Her son's health problems were severe, causing vocal cord paralysis and swallowing dysfunction. He also suffered from muscle spasms and had to have a tracheotomy. Senator Howard Metzenbaum put the Mills family in touch with aspartame expert Dr. Louis J. Elsas, who concluded that Brandon had been exposed to high levels of phenylalanine. The child's developing brain cells would have been chronically exposed to 500-600 mg of phenylalanine. Karen filed a lawsuit. The Americans are more vociferous than we are, and our suspicions become legal charges.

In May 1985, Louisiana Democratic Senator Russell B. Long told a strange story to journalist Alex Constantine about the evils of NutraSweet. Long told journalist Alex Constantine a strange anecdote about the evils of NutraSweet: "I recently received a letter from a person I know very well and whose speech is always perfect. She told me that she had been dieting and using aspartame drinks. She found that her memory was fraying and she felt that she was losing it completely. When she met people she knew intimately, she couldn't remember their names or even who they were."

This person was afraid of losing his memory. According to the senator, someone suggested that he stop taking NutraSweet, and soon after, his memory returned. If this is true, it's better than testing aspartame on lab rats!

According to Dr. Betty Martini, a woman named Cori Brackett ended up in a wheelchair after she stopped using aspartame. She had a brain injury she said was related to a lifetime of drinking diet drinks. After eight months of abstinence, the lesion disappeared. The same thing happened to Ermelle Martinez, also in a wheelchair. Mary Nash Stoddard suffered from cramps and pain so severe that she considered committing suicide. She saw six specialists for all of her pain, which mysteriously ended when she stopped drinking diet and consuming NutraSweet products. She spent a lot of money to find out if aspartame could be the cause of her problems. In the end, she indicted aspartame in its recommended baking use for diabetics. The NutraSweet representative, stated, "It is well marked that our products contain phenylalanine, those who cannot metabolize it well should know that [...] We can just teach others to cook well with aspartame." Mary Stoddard's husband died at age 42 of a brain tumor. Probably a coincidence. Since then, this journalist has been giving lectures, speaking out in the media and comparing the harmful effects of aspartame to those of cigarettes. The woman who used to use sweeteners in which she had blind trust, declares today: "How many spoonfuls of Equal does it take for it to cause a tumor of the pancreas or the liver? The answer is that I don't know, because it's a long-term effect... I saw the result on my youngest child who started suffering from migraines when he started drinking Crystal Light. He also had symptoms of a heart attack..."

She also reports that, while doing a story on airplane pilots, one of them told her that he had been having frequent headaches in flight for the past three years. When he stopped putting Equal in his coffee, the headaches stopped. It was pointed out to the reporter that millions of people drink diet beverages without these effects. Fibromyalgia, lupus, chronic fatigue did not exist before, she answered, nor so many psychological disorders in children, nor so many brain tumors. This is of course not a proof. In medicine or in criminology, you have to find the real culprit and *cold cases* take time to be solved. But prevention would undoubtedly help to avoid this kind of testimony.

Sometimes you might think you're in a contemporary play, like Molière, where "imaginary experts" make fun of real patients...

4 - ASPARTAME, BRAIN, ALZHEIMER :
FOR THE USE OF THE MEDICAL PROFESSION

Forgive the reader, but this chapter, which leads us to reflect on the "detail that kills" in a small way, is more for the medical profession. It is about the protein that is essential for stabilizing cells, especially the neurons in the brain. In the case of many diseases called "tauopathies", the most famous of which is Alzheimer's disease, Tau proteins aggregate abnormally and would be at the origin of neuronal degeneration. We asked Professor Narbonne about the link between aspartame and Alzheimer's disease. He explains the cerebral disturbances due to the metabolites of aspartame. His scientific arguments are addressed more to professionals in the field, but as diabetologists still prescribe E951 and are likely to believe him, the text remains in its entirety :

"Recently a link has been suggested between formaldehyde and Alzheimer's disease, shedding new light on the chronic effects of methanol. A first study concerns a chronic exposure of young macaque monkeys to a diet containing 3% methanol. This diet leads to a decline in memory functions that persists six months after the end of exposure. These functional alterations correspond to an increase in phosphorylation[82] of tau proteins in the cerebrospinal fluid during methanol exposure as well as an increase in aggregates of phosphorylated tau proteins and amyloid

---

82. Phosphorylation is the addition of a phosphate group that is transferred to a molecule or protein.

plaques[83] *in four brain regions identified postmortem: frontal, parietal, temporal lobes and the hippocampus. Tau proteins ensure the cohesion of microtubules constituting the skeleton of neurons and their synapses. This concordance between biochemical disturbances and functional disorders is consistent with a causal relationship. A study of the same protocol in mice (a 3.8% methanol diet for six months), showed an alteration of spatial recognition and olfactory memory. The immuno-histochemical study of the brain showed an increase in the phosphorylation of Tau proteins in the hippocampus and an increase in apoptotic processes*[84] *in more than 10% of neurons. In contrast, no amyloid plaque deposition was observed. This difference between rodents and primates could be explained by the differences in formaldehyde metabolism already reported. Two additional in vitro studies on embryonic cerebral cortex neurons and on mouse neuroblastomas*[85] *show that formaldehyde, but not methanol or formic acid, induces microtubule disintegration and hyperphosphorylation of Tau proteins. Obviously, we are not faced with the demonstration of a direct link between aspartame and Alzheimer's disease, but with a possible mechanism increasing the suspicions of neurological effects of aspartame that should be taken into account in the setting of safety factors. On the other hand, a recent study by Collison and his team investigates the chronic effects of a lifetime of aspartame exposure including the in utero period. When tested for spatial behavior, aspartame-treated males showed significantly longer acquisition times than untreated males. On aspartame-glutamate interactions, a study by G.M. Abu-Taweel and his team investigated the in vivo effects in mice of monosodium glutamate (MSG 8 mg/kg) and aspartame (ASM 32 mg/kg) individually or in combination on cognitive abilities and certain biochemical parameters such as neurotransmitters or oxidative stress indicators in the brain. After an exposure period of one month, the animals showed a strong alteration of the cognitive responses and of the*

---

83. Amyloid plaques are protein aggregates of neurons. Beta-amyloid cuts off synaptic communication. These plaques are found outside the neurons and were studied by Alois Alzheimer at the beginning of the 20th century. They are also called senile plaques.

84. Apoptosis is a programmed cell death in response to a signal. (From the Greek *apo*, "away" and *ptosis*, "fall") It was demonstrated by electron microscopy in 1972.

85. Neuroblastoma is the most common extra-cerebral solid malignancy of the young child that develops from the sympathetic nervous system.

memory and learning capacities. Taken separately, the two substances do not alter the biochemical parameters of the brain but the combination significantly decreases the levels of neurotransmitters (dopamine and serotonin) and also induces oxidative stress.

The relationship between a mother who uses aspartame and her unborn child raises a fundamental question: does the fetus have a risk of being disabled? Still according to the toxicologist Jean-François Narbonne :

"Maternal consumption of aspartame leads to saturation of cord blood with excitotoxic substances that can induce alterations in the development of the fetal nervous system. Similarly, an alteration of the blood-brain barrier can increase the circulatory levels of excitotoxic substances in the brain. This is especially true for areas adjacent to the ventricular system. It is also worth noting the similarity of the effects attributed to maternal ingestion of aspartame and those of fetal alcohol syndrome. I will conclude by saying that the potential neurological effects of aspartame and its metabolites appear to be an important consideration in the assessment of immediate or delayed risks from fetal exposure. This is one of the important points raised by the GECU because it can have important consequences in terms of public health, in particular for children, who are therefore the target population along with pregnant women. We can wonder about the substitution of sugar by sweeteners in pregnant women to compensate for gestational diabetes. In fact, the frequent report of cognitive disorders, even if not retained as conclusive by the EFSA, is still to be put in relation with the evidence of an oxidative stress affecting the central nervous system, with an induced deficiency of the enzymatic protection systems, but also with modifications of the neurotransmitters. This concordance of neurological effects in animals with symptoms reported in humans even at relatively low doses should have been considered by the EFSA panel. The conclusions of the GECU were presented on February 8, 2013 (one month to evaluate the EFSA report) and can be summarized as follows: contrary to the final choice of the EFSA experts, the GECU recommends retaining a daily dose of aspartame in application of an additional classical safety factor to take into account the toxicological aspect. It is all a question of interpretation: in fact the fundamental point of divergence between

EFSA and ANSES is linked to the duality of the data constituting the scientific file of aspartame. We are facing a toxicological exception because the ingested product does not penetrate the body: only the metabolites formed in the digestive tract are absorbed. The problem of possible toxic effects is therefore linked to the individual effects of the metabolites, which are, moreover, very common substances that are found in the body from different sources, including natural sources. In fact the dossier is composed of two parts. On one side of the scale there are the human data which concern on the one hand the effects sought by epidemiological studies and on the other hand the kinetic data of the metabolites to which the effects are due. If we adopt a classic approach, giving priority to animal studies, including those carried out according to the OECD protocol and meeting the GLP requirements[86], we are moving towards a reduced ADI such as that proposed by the ANSES."

The neurosurgeon Russell Blaylock accuses glutamate and aspartame of being together providers of excitotoxins, but he is hardly interviewed on television. It is true that talking about the BBB (*Blood Brain Barrier) is* a challenge and requires courage in the face of lobbies... The blood barrier of the brain is there to protect it from an excess of glutamate, aspartame, or toxins. But this barrier is not fully developed in childhood, and it does not protect all areas of the brain from toxins, which unfortunately allows the infiltration of an excess of aspartame and glutamate that act as neurotransmitters in the human brain. Their spread can trigger excessive levels of free radicals that drive cells to "suicide". They are healthy, and suddenly they die. Too much aspartame or glutamate in the brain causes excessive calcium ion invasion. Calcium in the gray matter is like a cerebral short circuit! According to Nicolas Blondeau and Catherine Heurteaux, from the Institute of Molecular and Cellular Pharmacology at the University of Nice: "Ischemic accidents (organ damage) and epileptic seizures are among the major causes of neuronal death. Unlike probiotics (for life), excitotoxins are pro-lethal... And obviously it doesn't take "kilos" to harm our brain.

---

86. *Good Laboratory Practices*: " Bonnes pratiques des laboratoires ".

5 - Excitotoxicity and Other Diseases

E951 is made of phenylalanine (50%), aspartic acid (40%), and methyl ester (10%), which is transformed into methyl alcohol - or methanol - and several other neurotoxic and carcinogenic products resulting from their degradation either by metabolic transformations occurring in the body, or by the exposure of the product containing aspartame to a temperature higher than 30°C This was the first core sample required before any reflection. Let's now go back to the tracks, coincidences and information, to cross-check some facts. By changing the angle, one ceases to have a flat vision and the reflection takes volume.

In 1957 two British ophthalmologists, Lucas and Newhouse, had observed the toxicity of glutamate by noting the destruction of neurons in the inner layer of the retina of newborn mice fed with monosodium glutamate. About ten years later, the American Olney discovered that this phenomenon was not limited to the retina, but concerned the whole brain, and it was he who named this phenomenon "excitotoxicity". Excitotoxins destroy neurons, explains Dr. Russell Blaylock, American neurosurgeon and nutritionist, in his book, *Exitotoxins: The Taste that Kills*. But glutamate and aspartame together are more threatening in the presence of other additives and dyes. They cause an excessive invasion of calcium ions in the brain. We imagine that certain chronic neurological diseases are caused by long-term exposure to excitotoxins. The exposed brain suffers, then certain pathologies appear: multiple sclerosis or similar symptoms, memory loss, hormonal problems and neuro-endocrine disorders, hearing loss, epileptic seizures, Alzheimer's disease, Parkinson's disease, hypoglycemia, dementia and brain damage. All of these are caused by excitotoxins. So aspartame has its share of responsibility. The list is close to a hundred cases and yet specialists cannot find the cause of these diseases when they appear abnormally early. It is difficult to say when aspartame is responsible and at what rate. But there are drugs where aspartame is contraindicated, which is a clue to the risks for infants, children, pregnant women, the elderly or those with chronic health problems caused by excitotoxins.

All the by-products of aspartame are addictive with an intense withdrawal phenomenon for heavy aspartame users, when they try to stop using it overnight. Aspartame causes an addiction, but is it a drug? The Pentagon was interested in it, considering that it was a biochemical weapon.

One of the common complaints among people suffering from the effects of aspartame is memory loss. Coincidentally, in 1987, Searle, the original manufacturer of aspartame, before it was bought by Monsanto, was already researching a drug that could combat memory loss caused by damage from excitotoxic amino acids. We have gone from the chemical formula of aspartame to the brain damage caused by excitotoxins that attack neurons.

The alarms are there, but the fire department arrives after an old fire. In this case, it's the "brain" house. Dr. Waickman, a pediatrician specializing in allergy and immunology, Dr. Hain, specializing in forensic pathology, and Dr. Roberts, a diabetes specialist, kept alerting the world, which never put out the fire, i.e., the manufacture of additives harmful to health.

Now here is a very interesting cross-sectional story. Psychiatrist Ralph S. Walton discovered that aspartame lowers serotonin (a monoamine, a neurotransmitter in the central nervous system, which causes depression when it drops). He realized this during the emergency hospitalization of one of his patients for severe depression. The patient suddenly suffered from epileptic seizures, which was clinically impossible. When asked what had changed between his home and the hospital, the man replied that at home he always took his tea with aspartame, and that in the hospital he was deprived of it! This lead proved to be more than indicative. As early as 1985, the psychiatrist detected nervous breakdowns in other patients due to the sweetener. No absolute proof, but a bundle of presumptions.

As a precaution, knowing that the brain cells have not been prepared for simultaneous and hidden invasions, we could prevent many patients from suffering from disorders whose origin they do not know. For the last two or three years, life expectancy seems to have decreased for the first time. Could it not be that diet, stress and the chemical components of our food are the cause? The role of sweeteners cannot be ignored. In 1995, an American study based on data from the National Cancer Institute suggested a possible relationship between the increase in the frequency of brain tumors in humans and the consumption of aspartame. This increase can also be attributed to cell phones, so studies should be comparative.

In 2005, 2006 and 2007, the European Foundation for Oncology and Environmental Sciences in Bologna published the results of studies on rats, whose conclusions suggested an increased incidence of lymphoma, leukemia and other types of cancer in animals exposed to aspartame. She sacrificed thousands of rats to understand the impact of sweeteners on health. Despite a permanent *bashing*, Dr. Morando Soffriti, from the Ramazzini Foundation, kept informing EFSA, which continued to denigrate his work. Here is the answer given by the accused: "The results of our studies show that aspartame, administered at variable doses, causes a statistically significant dose-related increase in lymphomas/leukemias and malignant tumors of the renal pelvis in female rats and malignant tumors of the peripheral nerves in male rats. These results demonstrate that aspartame is a carcinogen, capable of inducing tumors at doses below the acceptable daily intake of 40 mg/kg body weight in Europe, and 50 mg/kg in the U.S."

He was told that he had not demonstrated anything... In an interview given to Thierry Souccar, Soffriti says: "If something is carcinogenic in animals, then it should not be added to food, especially if there are so many people consuming it." This doctor, who has spent nearly 30 years studying potential carcinogens, was, with his team, one of the first to show that vinyl chloride, benzene, and the notorious formaldehyde are carcinogenic in an animal model.

Between politics and industry, is there any room left for the human, for humanity? Is it profit that leads the world and not ethics? Ethics are at half-mast, otherwise we would have really determined a dose without toxic effect designated as threshold dose[87] . But there will always be those in denial who do not care about the unresolved neurological problems. While Dr. Wurtman indicates that increased brain uptake of phenylalanine can cause seizures, the general public remains confident since "aspartame" products are available over the counter. Alcohol and cigarettes are harmful, but that is the choice of the consumer. Sweeteners are not officially suspected of anything, the manufacturers do not mention any risk, that is the difference!

Physician and journalist Marco Torres talks about collusion between sweetener manufacturers and the FDA, and then reports that 80% of the complaints filed with the Food and Drug Administration come from aspartame. The reports conveniently mention seizures, brain tumors, blindness, and even deaths. This is probably why French toxicologist Jean-François Narbonne responded as an expert to the global Diet Coke manufacturer who wanted his opinion: "I told them to withdraw this sweetener right away. There was at least one possible alternative right now for consumers: stevia, a natural product." This large group listened to him but did not call him back...

The American doctor Joseph Mercola added to the list of diseases probably linked to aspartame: Hodgkin's lymphoma and leukemia, explaining that man cannot fight against formaldehyde and formic acid. He claimed that *Diet Coke* products could contain up to 190 mg of aspartame. Coca-Cola's counter-attack to minimize the risks was this argument: a tomato juice contains six times more methanol than an aspartame drink. Natural methanol may come from rotting tomato skins, but not from the tomato itself, otherwise it would only mean that the tomato juice contains additives... Further on, Dr. Mercola explains that "every cell contains structures called peroxisomes that can help detoxify methanol. It is these peroxisomes,

---

87. This threshold is called NOAEL: *No-Observed-Adverse-Effect Level* (or "maximum dose without observed adverse effect"). Conversely, LOAEL: *Lowest observed adverse effect level* is the "minimum observed adverse effect level".

found in large quantities in the kidneys and liver, that convert formaldehyde into toxic formic acid; for humans, it is this step that is dangerous, as formaldehyde is a known carcinogen that causes retinal damage, interferes with DNA replication and can cause birth defects. Peroxisomes do have a detoxification role, but they cannot do everything in genetic diseases where they are absent. And precisely, disorders occur when peroxisomes disappear, reducing the functions of many enzymes, such as peroxidases. Peroxidases are the enzymes that break down toxic peroxide compounds. Some disorders include Zellweger syndrome (genetic mutations), neonatal adreno-leukodystrophy (a rare neurodegenerative disease), Plecolic acidemia (an enzyme deficiency) and orphan Refsum disease. Some babies may be born without muscle tone, others with brain malformations, seizures, and eye abnormalities. There is no specific treatment, and these "disorders" are lethal... These rare diseases are not well known by caregivers. But according to Marie-Cécile Nassogne, a specialist in metabolic diseases at the Saint-Luc pediatric neurology department in Brussels, hyperphenylalaninemia has very specific symptoms. Apart from the absence of signs in the neonatal period of progressive cerebral intoxication, there are mental retardation, microcephaly, epilepsy, psychiatric disorders of the autistic type, as well as a particular mouse-like odor, pigmentation anomalies, etc. For these children, Dr. Nassogne proposes treatments "and especially not aspartame!!!", she says. ANSES talks about tolerable doses of aspartame, but makes it clear "that historically, the toxicity of amino acids has been understood through the study of metabolic diseases such as phenylketonuria or leucinosis." Leucinosis is a pre- and neonatal disease whose symptoms appear five days after birth with cerebral atrophy.

New orphan diseases have been progressing since the 1980s. In France, three million people are affected by rare diseases. About five new diseases are identified every week! The accepted threshold in Europe is one case of an orphan disease in two thousand. Aspartame may be suspected to be at the origin or in connection with some of them.

If we should not put everything on the back of his worst enemy, the investigation leads us however to the strange alert launched by *bodybuilders*. According to them "three grams of D-aspartic acid increases testosterone levels by 40%". On a forum called Muscle Power, users express themselves. The article of one of them deserves to be quoted in note[88] , respecting the anonymity wanted by its author. Let's imagine that a *bodybuilder* adds aspartic acid to his doping products, and he is sure to age softened and feminized.

As for phenylalanine, it is essential to remember that it is not synthesized by the human body. It is an aromatic amino acid precursor of adrenaline. It is found on sale as a neurotransmitter with "magical" powers, used for athletic performance. But beware, these products can only be used in case of deficiency and according to medical advice. However, they are sold over the counter on the Internet and in some stores not run by pharmacists! On children, it causes irreversible brain damage, it is forbidden to pregnant women. According to the site agro-media.fr, the denial of the effects of aspartame would hide multiple risks and there would be a link between the increase in the consumption of aspartame and the number of brain tumors, and "an increased risk of premature births for pregnant women consuming aspartame, a greater occurrence of

---

88. *"Do not use a D-aspartic acid supplement until you read this article, you could be doing more harm than good! D-aspartic acid is all the rage right now in sports supplements. It has the potential to boost testosterone in multiple ways, but there is a hidden danger that people all need to know about using this popular bodybuilding product. That danger is increased* estrogen *production through aromatase. Aspartic acid is analogous to sodium D-aspartate and N-methyl-D-aspartic acid. They are becoming very popular with "bodybuilders" looking to increase their testosterone to the highest levels. However, this has a very ugly side effect that could make this innocent supplement the devil in disguise. It acts on an enzyme essential in testosterone production [...] It has been shown in human studies that D-aspartic acid can give an increase of about 30% in testosterone production! That's amazing for an all-natural product, but one that stimulates testosterone [...] Aromatase is a nasty enzyme that is responsible for converting testosterone to* estrogen *in the body. This is what robs the bodybuilder of the robust effects of testosterone and alters the balance of hormones. As we age, we produce even more aromatase and that explains why you see men get fatter, flabbier and flabbier as they age! Unfortunately, it seems that the "Holy Grail" of vitamin D-aspartic acid supplements can actually cause the body to produce more aromatase. It has been shown in the literature that D-aspartic acid can increase levels of testicular aromatase..."* It should be explained that aromatase is an enzyme that is part of the Cytochrome P450 superfamily, whose function is to aromatize androgens and thus produce estrogens. In girls, too much of it causes early puberty. For more information, see the *Guide de chimie médicinale et médicaments* by Serge Kirkiacharian (Lavoisier 2010).

stroke and heart, hepatotoxicity highlighted in rats by an Indian study. Thus, the long-term consumption of aspartame would lead to hepatocellular damage and changes in the antioxidant capacity of the liver.

Alarming studies are not considered convincing, whereas the first studies suspected of fraud are. The consumer remains in the dark, unaware of the risks he is taking, even if he thinks he is informed. Regarding the toxicity of formaldehyde, the opinion of the French Agency for Health Safety, Environment and Work dates back to 2004. However, formaldehyde is used in glues usually used in the building industry, a preservative and fixative known to pollute the interior of our homes. The AFSSA had been contacted in 2005 for some veterinary products containing it. Requested reports were delivered in 2008. This product alone can cause cancer of the nasopharynx in humans. Here is what the INERIS (Institut national de l'environnement industriel et des risques) says in its final report[89] concerning lethal effects: "No threshold could be determined due to qualitative and quantitative insufficiency of experimental data and the absence of data in humans. Regarding thresholds for irreversible effects, the data currently available in the literature do not allow the evaluation of irreversible effects induced by formaldehyde."

This is where the problem lies. On the one hand we are alarmist, on the other we are careless. Is there or is there not a health risk for the world's population, in priority for pregnant women, to ingest E951?

---

89. Ministère de l'Écologie et du Développement durable, Ministère de la Santé, de la Famille et des Personnes handicapées: Report by Blandine Doornaert and Annick Pichard, Direction des risques chroniques, Unité d'expertise des substances chimiques (ETSC).

NUMBERS AND CITIZENS TALKING

1 - Deepening of the subject and controversies

In a curious flashback, the numbers collide. In 1985, 600 alleged victims joined forces as Aspartame Victims and Their Friends, Inc. in Washington, D. C., with the Community Nutrition Institute, a Florida-based consumer group, claiming that human harm would be proven. C., with Community Nutrition Institute, a Florida-based consumer group, proclaiming that human harm would be proven. Young Dr. Frank Young of the FDA did the job again. The three judges were Mikva, Edwards and Starr, just as the FDA was about to approve aspartame in carbonated drinks...

Judge Abner Mikva wrote to the Court of Appeals. Prior to the results and decisions, the GAO (General Accounting Office) issued its report on July 16, 1987: the FDA had followed its own internal and external procedures. Sixty researchers had stated their confidence in aspartame, but the GAO could not assess whether the sweetener was safe or not. The question remained unanswered and then the use of aspartame skyrocketed. According to FDA estimates, it was necessary to limit the use of aspartame to three coffees or three teas per day, with a maximum dose of aspartame... But these last jolts to protect public health were no match for the very low price of sweeteners and their fantastic sweetening powers. In 2016, here are some figures that could be put into perspective:

Acesulfame **potassium E950**. Sweetening power: three hundred times sugar. Sold at 760 dollars per ton.

Alitame E956. Sweetening power: two thousand times the sugar. Between 2 and 5 dollars per kilo.

Aspartame E951. Sweetening power: two hundred times the sugar. Was sold at 1 dollar per kilo for a purchase by the ton. Today, it is sold according to quality from 10 to 22 dollars. On a Chinese site the ton is at 14 100 dollars.

Cyclamate E952. Sweetening power: thirty to forty times the sugar. Was sold at 13 euros the kilo.

Neotame E961. Sweetening power: between seven thousand and thirteen thousand times the sugar. Between 30 and 80 dollars per kilo.

Saccharin E954. Sweetening power: between three hundred and five hundred times the sugar. Per ton: 5 000 euros, and 8 or 10 euros per kilo.

Stevia (steviol glycosides) E960. Sweetening power of thirty to forty-five times sugar. Between 40 and 220 dollars per kilo.

Sucralose E955. Sweetening power: six hundred times sugar. 10 dollars per kilo.

Sugar: in France the price collapses. Sale from 0,89 euro the kilo.

Tagatose E963. Sweetening power: 30% less than sugar. Average price per kilo: 26 euros.

Thaumatin E957 natural or chemical. No price displayed. Sweetening power: two thousand to three thousand times the sugar.

No one compares these prices to the cost of health care, yet aspartame can cause type 2 diabetes. However, here are the figures given by the High Authority for Health: for all diabetics combined, the average annual reimbursement was estimated in 2007 at 5,300 euros per person. The amount of reimbursements increased with age, reaching 8,700 euros for people aged 85 and over. The amount reimbursed for antidiabetics increased by 5.9% in 2009 compared to 2008, reaching 716.9 million euros. And if we talk about the secondary diseases accelerated by diabetes, because it has just been proven that high blood sugar levels reduce cognitive faculties, then we must mention the 850,000 French patients suffering from Alzheimer's for a total cost of 5.3 billion euros per year... So, the savings made by the sweetener manufacturers cause colossal health expenses.

However, it was known as early as March 1972 that rats autopsied at Searle showed questionable pathologies, and less than ten years later, this monograph was a thing of the past. This kind of cover-up takes "centuries" to resurface because the truncated results of yesteryear remain valid. The toxic effects have not been brought to light. Who is going to sue the Searle lab for removing tumors from animals to mask the effects of its magic powder? Who can claim to understand what the labels on our everyday consumer products do not say?

Rumsfeld made part of his fortune with Searle and a discovery that should have been left on the shelf: aspartame. In the 1977 *Wall Street Journal,* he claimed that he acted "like a watchdog, for the sake of Searle's reputation," to ensure that no test was falsified. In vain, Senator Howard Metzenbaum participated in the hearing on NutraSweet: Health and Safety...

The names, the facts, fit together like in a film noir scenario.

An internal report on aspartame-related guinea pig disorders was signed by John S. Arnold, David M. Erspamer, both investigators, Dr. Jean Taylor, toxicologist, Dr. Leonard Friedman, biochemist, Jerome Bressler, team leader. Each page is marked "Searle Laboratories. Div. G.D. Searle & Co, Skokie, Illinois 60076". A document from the *Wall Street journal,* available on the Internet, puts Searle's interests into perspective and exposes the old lies[90] of the so-called *Big Pharma.*

The factory was in Skokie. In Skokie, they did everything from research to cures to forged documents. Skokie was a nice little town and Searle moved there. In 1963, the railroad tracks stopped right in front of the labs. In the 1970s, there was a huge fire in the labs. Precisely, on June 27, 1977. Loud explosions were heard. Seven firemen were hospitalized because of smoke inhalation. It was the most dangerous fire according to the 100 Skokie firefighters who arrived at the scene of the explosion: the laboratories located at 4901 Searle Parkway. It was the year Searle (now Pfizer[91]) approved dry

---

90. See Appendix 3.

91. Pharmacia Corporation is owned by Pfizer (Skokie). The company was created by an agreement between Monsanto/Searle and Pharmacia & St. John. Pfizer Inc. and Pharmacia Corporation unified their companies in April 2003.

aspartame under the name NutraSweet. The year Jerome Bressler reported on the astounding tests done in situ. It was also in June 1977 that Donald Rumsfeld was appointed president of the Searle Group. In Skokie, a strategic suburb of Chicago, many people worked at G.D. Searle before being linked to intergovernmental affairs or environmental protection. The prosecutor in charge of the criminal investigation against Searle resigned from his position before joining his law firm. In 1977, evidence of conflict of interest, ambiguity and pressure forced William Conlon, the last investigator, to give up. Journalists don't always have time for long term memory, and those who take too much aspartame lose it, so the case was quickly watered down. Donald Reagan appointed Arthur Hull Hayes, a former Pentagon researcher, to head the FDA, the same man who organized the panel in response to the controversy in 1981.

Monsanto bought Searle for $2.7 billion. Rumsfeld and John Robson only changed the host, which was actually the same one. All gained in strength and strategy[92] . Robson went from Searle to Pharmacia Corporation (Monsanto) before running Exide Corp, and becoming a banker, politician, and science start-up booster. Nicholas Filippello, vice president of Monsanto, quietly waited for FDA approval for the use of aspartame in baked goods. In October 1988, the approval was granted and the Skokie site continued to grow.

In Atlanta, home of Coca-Cola, in 1984, the Center for Disease Control, Nutrition Division, issued a 146-page report in November evaluating 592 consumer complaints related to aspartame. 75% were from women. Ninety-four percent were white, 77 percent were between 21 and 60 years of age, the youngest being 4 months old, the oldest 77 years. The recognized symptoms were: aggressive attitude, disorientation, hyperactivity, excitability, numbness, loss of perception and memory, liver failure, water retention, cardiac arrest, suicidal tendencies, seizures, headaches, mood swings, death. According to industry experts, the symptoms were not related to aspartame but to consumers in poor health. Aspartame has been indicted by *class actions* in the United States. Monsanto has not manufactured aspartame since the year 2000.

---

92. See the January 19, 1985 *Chicago Tribune* article to follow the transactions.

And in the "authorized" circles, they still make fun of the studies of the Italian Ramazzini Institute and those of Abdel-Salam on the cognitive disorders which say that the ADI should be fixed at 20 µg/kg/d, that is to say two thousand times less than the current one which is 40 mg/kg/d[93].

We cannot go back to the past, but deal with the present. Sponsoring and lobbying always block certain inconvenient truths. They sometimes give themselves a good conscience with the professionals of the profession. For example, there is a photo showing the prize awarded in 2009 to a nutrition researcher at Inserm, in "complete independence" from Ajinomoto by Ajinomoto[94]. Let's be fair, not all Ajinomoto awards are focused on aspartame... But what an irony, "Professor Bernard Guy-Grand of the nutrition department of the Hôtel-Dieu hospital praised the originality of Nicole Darmon's work: 'They give a good indication of the influence of economic constraints on behaviors and their contribution to malnutrition and obesity'."

The mission of EFSA, founded in 2002, was to inform politicians to make intelligent decisions about "risks associated with the food and feed chain". It was to be independent and transparent. However, in order to sell food products in Europe, companies must request authorization from EFSA, which assesses the risks and gives its approval or not. The thick files that are transmitted to it are protected by the commercial secret invoked by the food multinationals. A decree linked to the industries almost deprived French journalists of sensitive investigations... The journalist Élise Lucet had launched a petition against this project. Concerning health protection, independent studies are conducted after marketing in order to preserve the secret of a product. It is like giving a judgment

---

93. On the site sweeteners.org France: "A woman weighing 60 kilos would have to consume 280 tablets or 20 cans of low-calorie sweetened soft drinks every day of her life" to be at risk... (about sweeteners and the safety of the acceptable daily doses)

94. The jury of the prize was chaired by Professor Bernard Guy-Grand. The other members of the jury were Professors Luc Cynobar (Hôtel-Dieu, Paris), Marc Fantino (University of Dijon), Claudine Junien (Necker Hospital for Sick Children, Paris), Martine Laville (Édouard Herriot Hospital, Lyon), Éric Lerebours (University of Rouen) and Dominique Parent-Massin (University of Western Brittany)

before a fair trial has taken place. If aspartame has been known for decades, as far as its effects are concerned, EFSA has not been able or willing to commission really contradictory studies; in fact, it is up to the consumer to consider the risks or to accept the industrial studies on daily doses with closed eyes!

In 2006 and 2007, Dr. Morando Soffritti had asked for an urgent re-evaluation of the rules on aspartame consumption. EFSA rejected his study because it did not comply with OECD standards (nor with the standards of industrial laboratories). In 2009, after a new independent study against aspartame, EFSA had reaffirmed its position. The cause of this refusal: the choice of certain mice for the experimentation. Dr. Soffritti had tested aspartame from the fetal stage until death, and observed that the risk of cancer increased when exposure to aspartame began during gestation. This study was also rejected on the grounds that the cancers could have occurred spontaneously. To support its statements, EFSA cited five other studies: two funded by industry: Rhone Poulenc and Dow Agro Sciences, one summarizes the conclusions of a working group of ILSI, the other is signed by an academic and collaborator of ILSI: Alan Boobis, the famous toxicologist who says that aspartame is not dangerous, even in children's milk. For the record, he was not concerned about the dioxins found in Irish pigs. It is interesting now to have the feeling of Pr Narbonne on the positions of EFSA, because he was as a toxicologist at the decisive meeting of 2013:

"The public consultation of EFSA following its 2013 report, was to conclude with a meeting where all organizations or personalities disagreeing with the position of EFSA could come to present and discuss their arguments. This meeting took place on April 9, 2013 in Brussels. ANSES was represented by the director of the chemical risks department and by me as an expert of the GECU. The morning was dedicated to the presentation of the different positions of the "contradicts" while the afternoon was dedicated to the discussion of the different positions with the EFSA expert panel. Some interesting observations about the participants. The first was the strong representation of the industrialists who were accompanied by one of the most influential English toxicologists, Professor Renwick from the University of Southampton, whose opinions had always seemed to me to be scientifically founded (even if they could differ from mine) in the numerous European meetings he had led. On the other hand, several English toxicologists, declared opponents of aspartame, were present. The second was the low participation of the national health agencies, only the Italian and French agencies were present. For Italy again, the Ramazzini Institute was well represented. Finally, for the NGOs, only the spokesperson of the RES was present. During the morning, each speaker came to present his arguments showing his divergences or convergences with the interpretation of EFSA. I was in charge of presenting the GECU ANSES report illustrating the criticisms reported in our opinion. Several remarks were made on this session: the quality of the presentation of the Ramazzini Institute, the perfect convergence of the positions of the Italian and French Agencies insisting in particular on the neurological effects, but on the other hand the mediocrity of the presentation of the RES whose presentation was limited to the reading of a slide consisting of the simple copy of the press release in English published by this network. The main argument insisted on the carcinogenic character of aspartame and demanded that the ADI be set at a few micrograms. This poor presentation contrasted with the document "Analysis of the EFSA report" published by the RES containing several relevant criticisms that could have been exposed on this unique occasion, possibly reinforcing the arguments presented by the other participants. This minimalist attitude was confirmed in the afternoon, which was devoted to a wide-ranging debate between the morning speakers and the EFSA panel of experts. Animated, even very animated, discussions took place in particular with the representatives of the Ramazzini Institute refuting the lack of expertise and seriousness reproached by EFSA with solid arguments. The English toxicologists opposed insisted on the metabolic aspects and the representatives of the French and Italian Agencies put forward the neurological and developmental aspects. Here also two remarks: The first one on the interventions of Prof. Renwick regularly supporting the position of EFSA, refuting with a certain contempt the arguments of the opponents. The second was the non-intervention of the RES representative who could have supported some of the opponents' arguments, which were also reported in the documents published by the RES. This was all the more surprising as the RES was presented in the media as the only "independent" opponent of aspartame and complained vigorously that it had never been heard by EFSA. Finally, EFSA maintained its position by saying that the arguments presented had already been taken into account and discussed in the report and that the few recent data not taken into account in the EFSA report were not likely to decrease the ADI either. A reduction of the ADI by a factor of 10 would not have prevented the continued use of aspartame in diet products but would have had a limiting effect on the consumption of pregnant women and children, the most sensitive populations. Faced with this blockage and the obligation to continue to apply the European ADI, ANSES has continued its benefit/risk approach because it remains possible for national agencies to issue consumption recommendations that remain in the realm of subsidiarity. Thus, in January 2015, ANSES published an opinion on the evaluation of the nutritional benefits and risks of intense sweeteners, whose conclusion deserves to be quoted in full:

"In conclusion, no beneficial effect has been demonstrated to recommend regular consumption of IE (intense sweeteners) in adults and children. Moreover, the available data do not show the existence of a risk in occasional consumers. On the other hand, the epidemiological data currently available do not allow to completely rule out certain risks in case of regular and prolonged consumption. Therefore, for the general population, the overall consideration of potential nutritional risks and benefits does not justify the long-term use of ARs as a substitute for sugar, especially in beverages, which are the main vehicle for sugar. In this sense, both sweetened beverages and sugar-sweetened beverages should therefore not be substituted for water consumption."

What a painful soap opera. We would have liked the experts to agree on the effects of the excess of aspartame and glutamate in the blood plasma and on what these two products can cause at the level of neurotransmitters in specific cerebral areas. We would have liked something more than a "everything is fine, sleep, eat, drink, we take care of you". We would have dreamed of a neutral authority verifying the EFSA data. However, a press release of the RES (Réseau Environnement Santé) opposing aspartame dated February 18, 2013 says that the EFSA opinion violates the rules of ethics of expertise by rejecting recent scientific data. EFSA is an authority that is not restrained in anything, it leads! It declares on its website[95] all the good that is expected of it, but ethics too often stops where conflicts of interest begin. In 2015, according to her, glyphosate did not present any carcinogenic risk and her advisors belonging to the promoters of risky products were credible. Consider one of her advisors: Dow AgroSciences. This firm is associated with Monsanto to develop new products together. As in genealogy, it is good to know who is related to whom, what are the knots, agreements and paternities... Dow AgroSciences[96] presents itself as one of the world's leading research laboratories for crop protection and pest control products. But what does this have to do with aspartame? Dow and Monsanto were partners in the manufacture of Agent Orange, the defoliant used in Vietnam. Together they have created a GMO corn and are working on the genome of plants and animals. A conference sponsored by Dow AgroSciences and the Bill & Melinda Gates Foundation was held in California in 2013 and it was there that we learned that Dow AgroSciences is in close relationship with EFSA on pesticides but also for food safety! The links are as close as between ILSI and EFSA. One can freely find joint conferences that confirm that the experts who should warn us are on the side of the "yield". If citizens' associations denounce the proximity between some EFSA experts and the industrial lobby, this has no impact because EFSA is independent from the European authorities; and only the European Parliament could question part of its financing. Unless strict rules are put in place to prevent any conflict of interest, nothing will

---

95. *"Food is essential for life. EFSA provides scientific advice to protect consumers, animals and the environment from risks associated with food. We provide independent scientific advice to decision-makers who regulate food safety in Europe. A set of core values guides EFSA's activities. We are committed to applying them in all areas of our work. We assess risks throughout the food chain, helping to provide Europeans with one of the highest levels of safety in the world."*

96. In France, the company's website states: *"Dow AgroSciences is a world leader in crop protection and improvement. These crop protection products improve the quality and quantity of the world's food supply and contribute to the food security of a growing world population."*

change. So the official story remains that of the chemical engineer who sucks his fingers and shouts, "Eureka, I found fake sugar." Thus, legends are built that mask reality. In fact, little is known about what happened to James M. Schlatter, born in 1942. Arthur Hull Hayes, on the other hand, passed away in 2010, having made it into the top 100 millionaires in technology during his lifetime. He was not only a soft drink businessman, but also a specialist from the military, close to Donald Rumsfeld. Now that things are coming together, we can better understand the original scenario. An investigation is based on verified facts and trial and error, so that congruent elements can be transformed from presumptions to definitive proof. So, let's replay the film with its opening credits and a few zooms before. Aspartame was first manufactured for Searle by Genex Corp in Rockville (a group specialized in DNA sequencing and GMOs, the chemical industry, linked to the Lilly laboratory) and purified in Baltimore. In 1987, Genex Corp sued Searle for licensing, fraud and violations of federal antitrust law. This led to the sale to St. Louis-based Monsanto Co. which had already made a joint venture with IG Farben[97]. The union between Monsanto and IG Farben resulted in Chemagrow Corporation. Monsanto remained linked to the Searle Group, so everything is in everything and vice versa... And now Bayer seems to be buying Monsanto. During the Second World War, the German group tested chemical agents; nerve gases with the Nazi Dr. Gerhard Schrader, who was then recruited by the U.S. Chemical Warfare Service. Otto Bayer died in 1982 after an industrious life as a chemist; it was he who obtained the synthesis of polyurethanes and polyol (glycol used to manufacture sweeteners). But he was not the owner of Bayer, just a namesake. Convicted of crimes against humanity at Nuremberg, and later dissolved, IG Farben, despite its dismantling, still has legal status. Monsanto had also created links with IG Farben's satellite companies before and during the Second World War. The American journalist Constantine

---

97. IG Farbenindustrie AG is the result of the merger in 1925 of three chemical companies: BASF, Bayer and Agfa. It was at the origin of the synthesis of methanol, the manufacture of antibiotics, Zyklon B and sarin gas. Dismantled for denazification in 1952 into twelve successor companies including Bayer, BASF, Dynamit Nobel, etc.

speaks of a "*Nazi's connection*" between Monsanto and the former pro-Nazi companies acquired. Many of the scientists hired in the U.S. weapons and chemical fields were former Nazis. Monsters old and new act without conscience. Today, Monsanto remains a pool of people close to power that Bayer wanted to buy for tens of billions. In this world of titans, no group really devours the other, but rather "enriches" itself. The sweetener business: aspartame, glutamate, saccharin, sucralose, is only one side of the iceberg, but the common philosophy remains the same: to sell. William Ruckelshaus[98], a former FBI boss under Richard Nixon, who was the first director of the Environmental Protection Agency, declared without blinking: "Monsanto should not have to vouch for the safety of *biotech food*." Phil Angell, one of the directors of communications, stated that "Monsanto's interest is to sell as much as possible, the FDA's job is to guarantee our products." William Ruckelshaus spent twelve years on the Monsanto management team associated with Ajinomoto. Present under Richard Nixon, Ronald Reagan and George H. W. Bush, he is now part of the Madrona Venture group of which he is a director (in strategy). The link between politics and the chemical industry never ends. With the BASF-Bayer-Monsanto merger, aspartame will be nothing but dust in this conglomerate, and many files will still be misplaced that EFSA will pretend to have read. The ostrich policy weighs on our destinies. It is up to us to be careful to assess the risks to our health.

---

98. See the Legal Information Institute website (law.cornell.edu) for his full resume.

2 - SCIENCE, CONSCIOUSNESS AND CITIZENSHIP

This last part testifies to the increase of certain diseases, while mentioning the part attributable to aspartame. In *60 millions de consommateurs* (n° 390), a file on the additives consumed without our knowledge, already warned in 2005, on the effects of E951: "Increase of brain tumors in the United States since the 80s". The article expressed a great mistrust towards the product suspected of causing epileptic seizures. But the "experts" authorized to explain were of a different opinion. For example, the question put to Mr. Gérard Pascal, former INRA and member of the "food additives" committee of AFSSA, was simple: why not ban carcinogenic products? Answer: "We must ban those that are genotoxic, but the others are only "promoters" of diseases...". In short, we were taking the risk of sacrificing the predisposed, by shortening their lives legally. And in the world, how many lives have been shortened? Under the pretext of health, we make sick those who absorb sweeteners. One thing is certain: formic acid does not occur naturally in our heads. It has been shown that ingestion of aspartame, especially with carbohydrates, can cause excessive levels of phenylalanine in the brain, even in people who do not suffer from the genetic disorder called PKU. Those who have taken in large amounts of aspartame over a long period of time have been found to have excessive levels of phenylalanine in their blood. Little by little, the investigation is leading to concrete evidence. An excess of phenylalanine in the brain can cause a decrease in the level of serotonin and this is what leads to emotional disorders, to depression. If this is still only the tip of the iceberg, small "CQFDs" - which are scattered all over the investigation - put the puzzle back together.

It is up to the medical profession to ask real questions and to take action on the subject. There are symptoms without any apparent cause: inflammation of the optic nerve, early ophthalmic problems, violent allergic reaction after mouthwash. Neurologists, doctors, dentists treat, but without linking symptoms with still unknown causes. There is no daily calculation between the amount of aspartame, neotame, advantame and other unreported sweeteners whose metabolites accumulate, so it is certain that doctors are unable to make a good diagnosis. They need proof! But there is evidence. In his testimony before the US Congress, Dr. Louis J. Elsas[99] demons-trated that high levels of phenylalanine in the blood can concentrate in parts of the brain and that this substance is particularly dangerous for infants and fetuses, and that phenylalanine is metabolized much more efficiently by rodents than by humans, which means that humans "digest" less well than guinea pigs. In the *Wednesday* Journal article "An aspartame Nightmare," a new piece of evidence supports this idea of overdosing: a man named John Cook began drinking six to eight diet drinks a day. His symptoms began with memory loss and frequent headaches, but this did not prevent him from becoming addicted to his "drug": diet sweet. He couldn't live without it. He developed an increased need for sweetened drinks. His physical condition deteriorated and he experienced severe mood swings and violent outbursts. Even though he did not have PKU, a blood test revealed an incredibly high phenylalanine level of 80 mg/dl[100]. He also developed abnormal brain function and brain deterioration. After stopping his aspartame consumption, his symptoms improved dramatically. This proves that one can have the symptoms of a disease without suffering from it, but only from an overdose of a product that causes the imitation of a known disorder...

---

99. Died in 2012, Prof. Elsas had worked on children with phenylketonuria through feeding with Dr. Bacosta , Steven Yannicelli, Rani H. Singh, Louis J Elsas II, Shideh Mofidi, and Robert D. Steiner.
100. In typical PKU, phenylalanine in the blood exceeds 25 mg/100 ml.

Another alert, some bipolar diseases are suspected to be triggered by aspartame. This does not prevent certain medications for mental or emotional disorders from containing it! Diets filled with aspartame can trigger psychiatric disorders. The psychiatrist Ralph Wolton described them in 2007. When no therapy works, he explains that it is time to suspect a chemical agent. Not enough serotonin: aspartame can be incriminated. In manic phases leading to hospitalization, Dr. Wolton noticed that people who consulted a psychiatrist often did so after an emotional break-up and that at this time of stress, their diet often changed, and often, in order to get back on track, the famous diet was imposed! Dr Ralph Wolton was convinced of the role of phenylalanine: "I was more and more convinced that aspartame could both trigger crises and exacerbate various psychiatric disorders. I presented a paper on such patients at MIT, at a sponsored conference... on dieting."

Vulnerable people are more vulnerable and suffer from the "allowed" doses. Fortunately, research continues. In 2006, Fabíola Azevedo Genovez de Lima Leme and Reinaldo Azoubel, in their work, talked about the effects of aspartame on rat fetuses. They used a 14 mg/kilo solution, given to pregnant rats for three days, either at room temperature or heated to 40°C. In the second case, the weight of the mothers as well as that of the placenta decreased. Statistically, the researchers saw changes in the exocrine cells of the pancreas. The pancreas secretes insulin - a hypoglycemic hormone - and glucagon, which is a hyperglycemic hormone, and also digestive enzymes. The pancreas weighs only 100 g, but it has "a thousand and one" essential functions. Lipases digest fats, amylase enzymes digest slow sugars. If the pancreas is affected by too much aspartame, then diabetes can occur. CQFD.

We now know that the transformation of aspartame in our body affects the pancreas, the intestines, the brain. The significant increases in phenylalanine levels are located in certain regions of the central nervous system[101]. In the end, it is as if there are two control stations: the brain and the belly. What happens biochemically, neurologically, and even electrically in our brains is beyond

---

101. *Medulla oblongata* and *corpus striatum*.

us, and we can only see the impact of excess phenylalanine on it. Blaylock pointed out that this overdose could lead to schizophrenia or cause a stroke. Ironically, long-term overuse of aspartame can lead to accelerated sales of serotonin inhibitors and high consumption of antidepressants. The last studies made during eleven years by scientists of the Brigham and Women's Hospital in Boston, show that there is also a strong correlation between aspartame and renal degeneration[102]. Correlations do not make proof, and as long as there are no independent investigations, the FDA can serenely affirm that everything found on the Internet concerning aspartame is a bunch of *hoax busters* and *fake news*. But what if it was the other way around? What if the liars are just finding ways to answer inconvenient questions?

More and more brands are selling aspartame-free products for pregnant women because moms-to-be know: the best products are the ones that are safe. Meanwhile, many at-risk consumers are unaware of the excitotoxicity of glutamate and aspartame. Europe is behind in its fight against fake good products. The American consumer leagues are not shy in incriminating Coca-Cola, Pepsi-Co, Bayer, Danone, Wrigley, ConAgra Foods, Wyet, Nutrasweet, Altria Corp (Kraft Foods Philip Morris). These twelve companies have found themselves before the Californian courts for fraud and lies about *diet* or *sugar-free* products. These very powerful and marketing-savvy groups were accused of putting a neurotoxicant in vitamin products, beverages, and even in children's aspirin. The courageous neurosurgeon Russell Blaylock evoked with certainty the link between the absorption of aspartame and macular degeneration, blindness due to diabetes, glaucoma, resulting from an overdose of the incriminated product. The studies submitted to the plaintiffs' file also evoked damages linked to the testicles, the thyroid, and the ovaries. The plaintiffs were ordered to stop producing and selling aspartame[103]. We have missed a new American legislation. If by any chance the deception of sweeteners is revealed to its full extent, then

---

102. *Clinical Journal of the American Society of Nephrology* publication of 3,318 women who consumed aspartame sodas.
103. Source: National Justice League.

real, costly, comparative and unbiased investigations will take place. But without waiting for the verdict, it is time for health specialists to take up the subject! Because the destruction takes place slowly, progressively, without blaming excitotoxins and the massive entry of calcium ions into the cells. Calcium is by far the most abundant metal in the body. It is mainly found in the bones, of which it is an integral part. Normally, calcium is involved in muscle contraction through the calcium ion Ca2+ and is also found in the pipes in the form of deposits! In the brain, calcium ions play a role in synaptic transmission. But the pathology born of excitotoxins causes Ca2+ ions to activate enzymes, including phospholipases C; and it is these enzymes that degrade cellular structures: cell membrane, cytoskeleton, DNA. Since this mechanism is also likely to occur after a brain injury, there is always a doubt, not about the diagnosis, but about the cause. This is why it is never easy to accuse a single factor. One thing is certain with sweeteners, there can be a lack of blood flow called ischemia, followed by an accumulation of glutamates and aspartates in the extracellular fluid, all of which is aggravated by oxygen and glucose deficiency. This is called an ischemic cascade: the one that causes cell death. It is this sequence of biochemical events that involves excitotoxicity. We speak of cerebral calcification due to excitotoxins, when a tumor is discovered whose symptoms are: epilepsy, paralysis, sensory deficits, cranial hypertension, headaches, vomiting. While victims are unaware of this vast subject, specialists know that aspartame can cause spikes in the concentration of aspartate in the blood plasma, spikes that other specialists ignore or find harmless. More and more clinicians are convinced that a group of excitotoxins due to the glutamate and aspartame couple plays a crucial role in the development of several neurological disorders, certain endocrine disorders, neuropsychiatric disorders, learning difficulties in children, AIDS-related dementia episodic violence, Lyme borreliosis, hepatic encephalopathy, specific types of obesity, and especially neurodegenerative diseases such as amyotrophic lateral sclerosis (ALS), Parkinson's, Alzheimer's and Huntington's, as well as olivopontocerebellar degeneration. The medical language seems complex, but we have to put things into words. How can very good therapists treat without prior education in toxicology? Many diabetologists still believe that aspartame is perfect for their patients and that these are rumors, false accusations about it. The controversy is still not settled and consumers will not get away without being informed. But by whom?

3 - MAPS, FIGURES AND CROSS-REFERENCES

In the face of unintelligible figures and empty words, this chapter is essential. Aspartame and other sweeteners are consumed en masse and rule without our conscious choice. The diet industry is gorging itself and complexes are doing the rest.

What remains of the fraud charges? Vague memories. Yet the exponential curves of aspartame consumption have been in the United States as well as in Europe and the world. Accepted Daily Intakes (ADIs) fluctuate from country to country. At the Montpellier Toxicology Society, Dr. Hervé Nordman is the one who takes the lead, and without fear of showing his membership in Ajinomoto before affirming that the ADI of 40 mg/kg is good. He is more than optimistic: "A meta-analysis of all controlled clinical studies conducted with aspartame shows that we can expect a weight loss of about 0.2 kg per week. Over a year, this allows you to lose more than 10 kg [...] It is the competition that is the origin of the haro on aspartame but in the face of very severe attacks, its safety has never been questioned by the registration authorities, nor by food safety agencies around the world."

We would like to believe it! Fortunately, in 2011, only about one in five French people consumed aspartame-based products at least once a week, according to a study conducted by the CRÉDOC. But there are 53 million diabetics in Europe. Diabetes, especially type 2, now affects 5.9% of the world's adult population, 80% of which is in industrialized countries. The WHO has warned that the number of deaths due to diabetes will increase by about 80% in some regions of the world over the next ten years! This means that the share of the global budget allocated to diabetes care in 2025 will be between 7 and 13%.

Type 2 diabetes, quite low in 1980, has jumped dramatically, but without any incrimination against E951 or anything. Few questions, few answers. During the Bichat talks in September 2005, France Bellisle, from Hôtel-Dieu in Paris, and Adam Drewnowski, from Washington University in Seattle, stated: "For years, we have been hearing that the consumption of diet products would lead to a phenomenon of "caloric catch-up"; this is what has been called the "sweeteners paradox". These assertions end up being considered commonplace, when in fact they are scientifically unfounded."

Can we believe these two specialists who are often solicited by Nestlé, whose double language is full of ambivalence: on the one hand, Nestlé incorporates additives such as aspartame into its products, and on the other hand, through its Institute, it presents itself as a non-profit organization whose wish is to share scientific knowledge in order to contribute to the quality of life of everyone, throughout the world. The report of the Ministry of Agriculture and Fisheries of March 2007, when diet drinks had increased by 20%, with a doubling of the market in five years, made the point with the same style of evacuation of the controversy: "The belief that intense sweeteners stimulate appetite and food consumption has not been confirmed by research work, both in the laboratory and in the field. The 'sweetener paradox' does not exist."

But what is the cause of type 2 diabetes, if not junk food and "bad drink" for sedentary and stressed city dwellers? By simple common sense we could solve the problem of overweight. But slogans have a hard life and everywhere we find the same phraseology that would like to reassure. To really inform consumers, we need irrefutable proof. Let's try to see more clearly in the immense rebus of consumption and disease figures, to expose plausible links between sweeteners and diseases.

There were 857 million overweight people in the world in 1980, there were over 2 billion in 2015. Today nearly 7,000 deaths a day (more than 2.5 million a year) are related to overweight and obesity, obesity costing $2 trillion in 2012. The majority of obese people live in North America, parts of South America, Europe, Saudi Arabia and Australia.

The obesity map seems to be a strict reflection of the Alzheimer's disease map[104] around the world, both for low and high rates except in two Gulf countries in 2012. It also looks like a sister to the map of consumption of sweetened or diet drinks.

The biggest soda drinkers are: in first place, Mexico with 105.9 liters per year and per capita and in third place, the United States with nearly 100 liters. It should be noted that there are few cases of Alzheimer's in Africa and no excessive consumption of diet sodas. What jumps out are the superimposed graphs: the curves of E951 absorption, followed by those of diseases like Alzheimer's.

The world population was 1.74 billion in 1910, 2.519 billion in 1950, 5.279 billion in 1990, 6.085 billion in 2000, 7.058 billion in 2012 and 7.2 billion in 2014. Consumers of aspartame and sweeteners will continue to increase, obesity, profits and risks too. According to researchers Françoise Clavel-Chapelon and Guy Fagherazzi, women who consume diet sodas have an increased risk of diabetes compared to those who do not consume sweetened beverages, and they have a 60% higher risk of suffering from diabetes, compared to those who consume conventional sodas in the same amount. Conversely, according to AminoSweet Europe: "Obesity kills more people without sweeteners: in Europe alone, overweight and obesity would cause 70,000 new cases of cancer each year. Diet drinks have increased from 0 to 7,000 million liters from 1979 to 2009. And the Ramazzini Institute's claims have been refuted by health authorities." End of quote.

The consumption of diet drinks was up in 2012 by 19.3%. 8 out of 10 obese people in the world drink light...

And there would be no correlation!

Knowing now that Alzheimer's disease affects nearly 36 million people out of more than 7 billion, some imagine that this number will have doubled by 2030. In 1980, out of a population of 4.5 billion, there were 11 million Alzheimer's patients. For 9 billion, we should have found 22 million cases. In 2005, 26 million people were already affected by the disease. This means that the number of Alzheimer's

---

104. See Appendix 5.

patients is exponential (10 million in the EU-27 alone, including Turkey). And the forecasts for 2030 are that nearly 72 million people will be more affected by neurodegenerative diseases than others...

Alzheimer's and dementia cases are increasing less in Latin America according to the WHO. Europe is almost at the same level as North America and the data on the cost[105] are staggering: dementia cases are expected to triple by 2050.

If we compare the use of diet food and the increase in Alzheimer's cases in the world: the maps combined with statistics show that in countries where overweight has taken hold, aspartame is present, and it is absent in others. Researchers should get out their calculators to clarify these statistical comparisons. Comparison between countries with high consumption of *low carb* or too poor to buy it: the geographies also correspond. In the Netherlands (16.9 million inhabitants), the average consumption of light drinks is 22 liters per year, with 253,000 cases of Alzheimer's. In France, for 65 million inhabitants, we have gone from 57 liters in 2006 to 66 liters in 2011, while overweight has increased from 15% to 34%. Correlation or no correlation? In Canada, out of 35 million people, the figure is 35 liters of diet drinks on average per person and 105,600 cases of Alzheimer's. In the United States, out of 315 million inhabitants, when they reached 85 liters of diet drinks per year and per person, 5.5 million people suffered from Alzheimer's with 1,300 cases diagnosed per day. To be precise: 1 case out of 20 around 65 years old, 1 out of 10 after 85 years old. Total cost of neurodegenerative diseases in the United States: 200 billion dollars... The cost of the disease is rising sharply, more than 66%, while heart attacks are falling, minus 13%. Alzheimer's cases are expected to double every 20 years. Orphan diseases are expected to follow...

China sees the number of obese children increasing. The percentage of Alzheimer's patients has also increased dramatically over the last twenty years. And if we compare the continents that are hungry and those that eat too much, we see that diet drinks and obesity affect the big cities more than the countryside.

---

105. Appendix 6.

The vertiginous phenomenon of urbanization that Africa is undergoing today predisposes its population to Alzheimer's disease in the years to come. This sad health forecast was revealed by Professor Christian Giordano, former professor of neurology in a medical science university in Côte d'Ivoire and also the father of neurology in that country. Three epidemiological studies were conducted in French-speaking Africa: in Djidja (Benin), in Bangui (Central African Republic) and in Brazzaville (Congo), in order to estimate the prevalence of dementia in subjects over 65 years of age and to study the risk factors for these conditions. These studies, using the door-to-door method, screened approximately 500 subjects in each area with the *Community Screening Interview for Dementia* and the "five words" test. The prevalence of dementia was low in rural Benin (2.6%), whereas it was higher in the cities of Central Africa (8.1% in Bangui and 6.7% in Brazzaville). This is the only known lead revealed by the excellent 2010 thesis (University of Limoges, doctoral school on environmental sciences, Faculty of Medicine, Institute of Genomics, Environment, Immunity, Therapeutic Health) defended by Maëlenn Mari Guerchet. She answered my question: "It is certain that food consumption and eating habits are changing in Africa, as in many developing countries. Unfortunately, we have not conducted very extensive studies on the link between these factors and the occurrence of dementia. On a purely personal level, I was surprised by the high consumption of soft drinks. The prevalence of neurodegenerative diseases in Africa is probably not as low as was thought a few years ago, it is true. However, we have not yet been able to demonstrate the involvement of dietary factors. Our latest studies were conducted in urban and rural areas of two central African countries, with a dietary investigation."

As she points out, there are few studies on diet in Africa. However, the two curves of obesity and Alzheimer's disease follow that of soda and *low carb* consumption...

The promoters of aspartame deny any responsibility. AminoSweet simply refutes the accusation of aspartame-induced miscarriages. At Coca-Cola, they deny that diet soda is fattening, but the CEO of Coca-Cola North America, Katie Bayne, boasted that she only drinks the brand's sweetened beverages all day long. Coca-Cola denies that the increase in multiple sclerosis (or similar symptoms) is linked to Diet Coke, as does the European Food Information Council, for whom this is an unfounded inference. Health Canada adds "unfounded" to all other accusations related to aspartame. If it is such a good product, why is there a higher percentage of Alzheimer's cases or early Parkinson's cases in countries that use it? And can we add the percentage of strokes increasing?

As for toxicological analyses and dosage issues, things are difficult to compare. At the experimental level, rats are a hundred times less sensitive to methanol than humans. So no study is really serious if we take it as a reference. Marc Resch, from Montpellier, made a simple calculation: the ADI for aspartame is 40 mg/kg, but if the daily dose is calculated with the NOAEL (*No-observed-adverse-effect level*) of the rat, the human dose would be a hundred times too high!

What is the balance between economy and health? Is it not tilted in the wrong direction? It is up to consumers to come to their own conclusions. In France, there is article L. 121-1 of the Consumer Code which punishes misleading advertising, it is the only existing text that can be used. According to this article L. 121-1 issued from the law n° 2008-776 of August 4, 2008:

I. - A commercial practice is deceptive if it is committed under any of the following circumstances:

(1) when it creates confusion with another good or service, a trademark, a trade name, or another distinctive sign of a competitor;

2° when it is based on false or misleading allegations, indications or presentations concerning one or more of the following elements

(a) the existence, availability or nature of the good or service;

b) the essential characteristics of the good or service, namely: its substantial qualities, composition, accessories, origin, quantity, method and date of manufacture, conditions of use and fitness for purpose, properties and expected results of its use, as well as the results and main characteristics of the tests and controls carried out on the good or service.

II. - A commercial practice is also misleading if, taking into account the limitations of the medium and the circumstances surrounding it, it omits, conceals or provides unintelligible, ambiguous or untimely material information or fails to indicate its true commercial intent if it is not already apparent from the context.

Deceptive commercial practices are punishable by the penalties provided for in the first paragraph of Article L. 213-1:

Any person, whether or not a party to the contract, who deceives or attempts to deceive the contracting party, by any means or procedure whatsoever, even through the intermediary of a third party, shall be punished by imprisonment of up to two years and a fine of up to 300,000 euros, or by one of these two penalties only:
(1) the nature, species, origin, substantial qualities, composition or content of useful principles of any goods;
(2) the quantity of the goods delivered or their identity by the delivery of goods other than the specific goods which were the subject of the contract;
3° either on the suitability for use, the risks inherent in the use of the product, the controls carried out, the instructions for use or the precautions to be taken.
The amount of the fine may be increased, in proportion to the benefits derived from the breach, to 10% of the average annual turnover, calculated on the basis of the last three annual turnovers known at the time of the breach.

The *deadline* is approaching but nothing is happening, the manufacturers are not questioned, and never will be, because the law makers and those who are responsible for their respect do not prohibit sweeteners as toxic by their metabolites. The only answer to give is the refusal of the consumers to pay to be intoxicated.

A site worth visiting to learn more is aspartam-provings.info. It is a compilation in English, signed by Richard Bocock (London), on this story which is coming to an end. It contains a very old but very important piece of information: the use of metrazol, an old drug tested against schizophrenia by the CIA after World War II and also for torture in Camp King in Oberursel (Taunus, Germany), an interrogation center initially created by the Nazis in 1933. In note 101, we learn that metrazol increases convulsions in animals fed with aspartame[106]. Aspartame is therefore totally contraindicated for epileptics according to the work of Professor Emeritus Richard Wurtman, whose work is located at MIT. This is what needed to be demonstrated.

Each piece of information is a small piece of the gigantic puzzle. Thousands more are lying dormant... The public debate must therefore be constantly nourished. This positive attitude would allow the idea of prevention to make its way.

To demand the most scientific information and to make it educational through a policy free of lobbies is a challenge, but a particularly useful one for health and the reduction of disease costs.

How long will it take the train of progress without conscience to stop? Much more than two generations are usually necessary. Unless Russian roulette becomes apparent and the population panics in the face of commercial cynicism. One of the promoters of aspartame keeps getting awards: Monsanto, not to name it, gets awards, including the World Food Prize, received on October 17, 2013. This *World Food Prize*, presented as a Nobel Prize for food, was awarded to the vice-president of Monsanto, as well as to a member of the Syngenta group and to Marc Van Montagu, a Belgian scientist who is part of a powerful European pro-GMO lobby (European Federation of Biotechnology). Monsanto, whose charter is "Integrity, transparency, dialogue, sharing and respect", has imposed its *Monsanto Protection Act*, which places it above the law by a discreet amendment slipped into a budgetary law for agriculture, signed by Obama... It is up to the citizens to create the "Healthy Products Award" and perhaps then aspartame, advantame, neotame, saccharine, glutamate, will disappear from canteens and homes.

But the good news is that the Chinese have a plant, *gotu kola, which* has been used in India for thousands of years and is believed to enhance brain function. Animal studies have shown that it improves nerve transmission by increasing the complexity of dendrites. And for Indians, good news too: studies have shown that *bacopa*

---

106. Read the report to EFSA made in 2013 by Dr. Lesley Stanley toxicologist, with all the pathologies studied: *Review of data on the food additive aspartame.*

improves short and long term memory. *Ginkgo biloba* may protect brain cells from free radical damage by improving blood flow and oxygen supply. Curcumin, an anti-inflammatory and antioxidant, increases the elimination of beta-amyloid. Powerful antioxidant and anti-inflammatory, curcumin seems to provide protection against Alzheimer's disease.

4 - The word must remain with the citizens

An amendment was presented by Senator Aline Archimbaud and her colleague Jean Desessard on behalf of the group Europe Ecologie Les Verts (EELV). Mrs. Archimbaud was present for an interview. What was not the case of some deputies or senators doctors media. The ecologists wanted to insert an additional article[107] concerning the sweetened drinks, but the debates were not to their advantage and took place in an atmosphere of dialogue of deaf:

The Chair: "Ms. Archimbaud, is Amendment No. 347 maintained?"

Mrs. Aline Archimbaud then addressed the Minister of Health on behalf of her constituents in an officially shared concern to put in place coherent policies. Thus, the concerned senators informed about the work of the ANSES working group on the evaluation of the nutritional benefits and risks of the consumption of intense sweeteners by the general population. But they were told to read the EFSA conclusion from February 2011, which stated that:

"The proposed taxation of this ingredient is also contradictory with public health objectives in the fight against chronic diseases such as obesity or diabetes. Indeed, many scientific studies have shown that intense sweeteners, aspartame in particular, can respond to certain current health issues by helping diabetics, limiting caloric intake and contributing to good oral hygiene. Aspartame contributes to reduce the sugar and calorie intake of the products in which it is used. The prevalence of overweight and obesity in France, as we have already discussed, now stands at

---

107. See Appendix 6.

French parliamentarians have been asking for a long time that at least a mention of risk for pregnant women, the fetus and young children be added to any diet product containing aspartame - in pure loss! Should we opt for an individual prevention, or a general information in the absence of "precious help" represented by aspartame?

In November 2012, the French Senate tried to tax aspartame... The idea was abandoned. But Aline Archimbaud, the senator from Seine-Saint-Denis, did not give up. Her commitment was simple: to represent the citizens and to oblige the public authorities to be enlightened regulators. She has been trying for years to tax drinks sweetened with aspartame, giving time to the industry to change its policy. But the proposed amendments have been knocked down and retracted, constantly running into the good old alibis. She explains her unsuccessful attempts: "I filed amendments in the Senate two years in a row, with the support of the ecologists in a draft financing of Social Security. In the 2013 and 2014 budget, I proposed a light taxation of aspartame to encourage manufacturers to use something other than this widely suspect product. It is time to introduce prevention trade-offs in the public health budget. We must stop the massive use of products that can have serious health consequences."

It could not be clearer. As a parliamentarian, this senator insisted on the fact that she had the privilege and the duty to alert her fellow citizens. Better than some journalists, she took the time and the means to document herself: "I had access to documents on a product that was banned, then marketed, then banned and marketed again in an extremely disturbing way. The Minister of

Health found that there were not enough arguments. In 1950, we knew that asbestos was carcinogenic. We had to wait until 1997 to ban it. There were one million deaths in France, linked to asbestos. However, for aspartame, there are alternatives and we propose to the manufacturers a time of adaptation. What I don't accept is this way of turning a blind eye, by saying that there are not enough studies to invalidate the EFSA's blessings. It is distressing to see that economic arguments are also used against a health argument. "I am a doctor, Madam, and if I tell you that it is not dangerous, it is because it is without risk. That's the kind of argument I hear. I told the Minister of Health that she was taking responsibility by refusing my amendments twice. I refused to withdraw them. Once and for all, the economic interests of pharmaceutical laboratories should be separated from the public interest, and whistleblowers such as Irène Frachon should be protected. I myself was attacked when I questioned the status of medical sales representatives, paid by the laboratories to objectively inform doctors. It is a somewhat schizophrenic situation to be judge and jury...".

Regarding aspartame and other chemical products of daily consumption, Aline Archimbaud proposes to stop relying on expert reports paid by laboratories, but to finance public studies that would provide more reliable data: "In France, despite some progress such as the Xavier Bertrand law, some links remain opaque. Monsanto is an extremely powerful firm. Such groups approach parliamentarians, invite them to lunches, but their attempts to approach them have no effect. In the face of casualness and pressure, there is the Blandin law which protects whistleblowers. When defending public health, there is not only curative, but also preventive action in the face of epidemics largely linked to lifestyle.

The bill was introduced in the Senate by Marie-Christine Blandin and her colleagues with the aim of completing the alert mechanisms in terms of health monitoring[108]. It is within this framework that

---

108. In particular by the creation of a High Authority of scientific expertise and warning by the protection of natural or legal persons launching a warning in sanitary and environmental matters or by the establishment of a warning cell in public establishments of an industrial and commercial or even administrative nature.

4 - The word must remain with the citizens

Senator Aline Archimbaud classifies the manufacture of aspartame, beverages and products made with aspartame. She praises the magazine *Prescrire*[109] which promotes independent researchers and not "ghost writers". She adds: "What is needed is a strengthened public research system that is not subject to pressure, and courageous parliamentarians. We are far from the goal, but we will continue. The first value is the respect of the general interest, which is not opposed to the economic interest, as people think. It is the role of politicians to mobilize consumers who have an enormous force, because they can become a powerful economic lever by boycotting aspartame. With a more expensive aspartame, manufacturers will find the alternative."

The special tax on aspartame did not see the light of day. The courage and representativeness of an elected representative cannot speak for the citizens. The senator's amendments were rejected. And the words of the then Minister, Mrs. Marisol Touraine, to fight amendment 23 *bis* concerning energy drinks were more than vague, except for their conclusion: "Mr. General Rapporteur, I understand the motivation of this amendment, but I would like to convince you that it is not necessary in view of the objective you set [...]. You can be sure that we share the same objective. I therefore ask you, Mr. General Rapporteur, to withdraw this amendment."

If the deputies, senators, ministers cannot take into account the desires and needs of consumers and voters, the latter must take charge themselves and appropriate all the information for themselves and their children. Light energy drinks exist and promote hyperalcoholization phenomena. *Binge drinking* sends kids to the emergency room. These drinks force the body to go and draw survival energy from the bones, and sometimes the heart stops... Some deaths have been recorded among the very young, due to this exhaustion that is provoked but not felt. But the industry does not panic for "so little". New amendments were proposed in November 2014, but to no avail. The minutes of the November 12 session can be found

---

109. The medical magazine *Prescrire* is not dependent on advertisers (pharmaceutical laboratories), yet it did not want to answer our questions about aspartame and obesity, as it had no records to provide.

on the Internet and can be summarized with this sentence: "it was difficult to go further, due to the lack of an impact study."

The one of November 22 reports laughter and an amendment not adopted after Jean-Claude Requier, senator of the Lot, has retraced the history. This was a failure... However, the right, then the left and the greens, all had once been in agreement on this real public health issue. When the union comes up against a renunciation from "higher up", nothing changes. What about the simplest morality? What to do to become a "consumer actor"? Keep informed, and sometimes directly on the big sites like the FDA, the ANSES, and look for scientific communications, compare, analyze, hoping that the journalists of earthenware are protected from the force of the lobbies of ironware.

In 2016, English MPs passed a tax on sugary drinks to combat obesity, but not on sweetened drinks. 28% of children aged 2-15 and 61.9% of adults are reportedly obese or overweight in England...

Betty Martini has chosen August 28 as World Aspartame Awareness Day. She is not the only one who wants products containing aspartame to mention it as a mandatory ingredient in human and animal food. The challenge is to convince the "believers" in aspartame of the dangers it may represent. It is a belief and not a medication. There are forms of food and pharmacological religions, common sense remains a compass. I hope that this investigation will have contributed to enlighten consumers, researchers, historians and journalists.

CONCLUSION

The human genius is to lead us generation after generation towards a more or less collective consciousness. Since prehistoric man, through exceptional beings such as Pythagoras for whom food was linked to the effort of mind and body, Leonardo da Vinci and Elisée Reclus, two notorious vegetarians, we are looking not only for energy to survive or live, but for an adequacy between what comes out of and enters our mouths: words and food. Words and food constitute us in a way. We are sometimes what we say and what we eat. Aspartame is not a part of the hygiene of life, it is not a progress like the cold chain, *but* a regression. Salt and sugar are natural preservatives, but as the late Jean-Pierre Coffe would have said, intense sweeteners are crap!

E951, a chemical substance among many others, modifies our metabolism and therefore our whole being. What if we did like Georges Perec who in his book *La Disparition* removed all the "E"? In reality, it is up to the industry to turn back the clock and return to gastronomy, to undisoriented taste and to respect for consumers. Nutrition is a barometer of our willingness to be landlubbers made of products from the land and the sea, with real nutrients that are essential to health. If light is heavy, then to live light, let's live healthy. It's up to the consumer to decide. But if he is addicted to a product, the industry will want to keep him as a client or patient. The latest news: PepsiCo has decided to reintroduce aspartame in its sodas in the United States after the commercial failure of new artificial sweeteners... The human guinea pig has become accustomed to artificial flavors. As for information on sensitive subjects such as aspartame, it turns out that it is not the citizens who decide, but the empires whatever they are: state, financial, etc. There remains the magnificent interstice of the freedom to think and choose without being too wrong. Clemenceau said: "Life is a chance to dare. To distinguish, to interpret what is. In the tangle of universal activities that blind us before enlightening us, the primitive effort of our understanding leads us astray in a forest of appearances" (*Au soir de la pensée*, 1927).

So let us dare to express our will to remain free to eat well, drink well and live well on such a generous planet! Let's be on our guard, because according to the American political scientist Zbigniew Brzezinski, in his book *The Grand Chessboard*, Europeans are increasingly admitting that in order to "catch up" they must become Americanized. Brzezinski coined the word *tittytainment* to define a "cocktail of mind-numbing entertainment and ample food to keep the world's frustrated population in good spirits." This advisor to many American presidents is part of the so-called Chicago school. His advice to the American power, to weaken Europe, by a junk food and a culture down. It is necessary to read Brzezinski before returning to the school of common sense, without waiting for the excuses of those who deceive us. In the face of lies, it is better to look for some saving and sincere truths. The word sincere comes from beekeeping and means "without wax", and therefore without cheating on the goods. It is up to us to make our honey from the flowers of truth...

It took me a long time to write this book. But "thank you" to all those who put obstacles in my way or let me go during the investigation, that only increased my will to clear such a complex subject and to have it published. My only goal is to share my investigation that others will enlighten with their knowledge.

A real big thank you to H. P., from the association La Règle, for his support during the scouting. To Professor Narbonne and Senator Archimbaud, to the late Claude Reyraud and his sharing curiosity, to the late Philippe Durrèche. To Luciano Melis, Georges Campero and Blandine Du Parc for their advice. To Michel Jacquemard for his support and his judicious remarks. To all the Max Milo team, without whom I would not have been able to share these chapters... Thank you, reader, for your curiosity.

APPENDICES

APPENDIX 1

As a doctor of pharmacy practicing in a pharmacy in Paris, I have always been concerned with the prevention of diseases induced by exogenous chemical factors present in our environment.

At my pharmacy counter, I had the chance to experience Henriette Chardak's fight to reveal the dangers of aspartame through this book.

The arrival of this book is a chance for each of us to become aware of the extent of the consequences that a chemical molecule can have on our health.

What if aspartame was just the tip of a huge iceberg?

How many toxic substances contaminate our daily lives and endanger our health? Are we surrounded?

What if aspartame was only the tip of the iceberg? How many toxic substances contaminate our daily lives and put our health at risk?

I remember the year 2004, my daughter was 8 months old, and at the counter of my pharmacy, I discovered, thanks to the revelations of one of my journalist clients, the presence of bisphenol A in baby bottles. She was appalled by her discovery and so was I.

I am a pharmacist in Paris and public health is a daily concern because I am too aware of the impact of each chemical molecule on our body and the fragility of our health.

At that time, baby bottles were made of polycarbonate. This material, polycarbonate, which is transparent like glass but virtually unbreakable, was made from a polymerization of bisphenol. Bisphenol is an endocrine disruptor capable of deceiving the various hormone receptors and causing consequences on physiological development.

This polymerization was not that stable over time. I then discovered how the bisphenol migrated from the polycarbonate into the milk, with temperature, wear and tear, and scratching. The older the bottle gets, the more it degrades. Surprised to discover that baby bottles could be toxic for babies, I decided to contact the manufacturers of the bottles I sold because I could not believe it. When I contacted them, the manufacturers answered that they knew it, but the European norms tolerated a threshold that should not be exceeded and they respected it. By testing a bottle over 50 uses, a reference brand was below the threshold limits. For a baby, 50 uses, that's one week of use. Another well-known reference brand also knew this and was preparing new bisphenol-free bottles for the coming months. I decided to put the glass bottles back on the shelf and to inform as many parents as possible.

But who is more at fault? Are the manufacturers at fault or are the standards set too low? It was not until a few years ago that Canadian consumer associations mobilized and set the world on fire. Bisphenol A was then banned in everything that was in any way related to babies. Everything had to be BPA-free. The problem is that today it is replaced by BPA-F, urethanes and vinyls whose harmlessness is not established but which are not banned.

We play cat and mouse. Now we are starting to see the bisphenol A disappear from the paper used for credit cards and receipts. But when I ordered the thermal paper for my printers and spoke with the distributor, he told me that in the paper without bisphenol A there is bisphenol B, which is even more toxic.

What to do? Who is in charge of checking all this?

How many products surround us and discreetly endanger us? How many people burn scented candles or incense while they give off toxic fumes, while others diffuse air fresheners and breathe them in all day in their car, with the windows closed, without suspecting that all this chemistry is not without danger? These luxury perfumes are sold at a high price and are deposited daily on our skin without any toxicity information.

These furniture manufacturers who offer prices so attractive that we are pushed to ignore the risks of formaldehyde, carcinogenic and responsible for respiratory irritation and headaches, present in the glue used to manufacture chipboard, and which will be released for several years in our apartments to the closest of the children.

Polyurethane, used in almost all mattresses, gives off toxic fumes that we breathe in all night.

By what means to take all these problems, have we not gone too far in this industrial freedom which does not hesitate to propose "super products" so innovative that we end up forgetting the sacrifices to make on our health.

I'm sure many are unaware of all these risks and would appreciate knowing about them, but what if everything is contaminated?! What if we end up having something to blame on almost every product? Does constant vigilance border on a form of paranoia that we would like to avoid?

How many Smartphone users abandon iPhones for Samsung because the SAR (the quantification of toxic wave emission) is much lower, I think that many know it but that Apple's communication is too seductive to give in to caution, besides no brand uses this argument to hope to increase sales. Are we ready to sacrifice what we want to buy to save our health or do we have to choose between health and the product?Why are all these toxic products now in our environment and why are the manufacturers not obliged to demonstrate the harmlessness of their products before marketing them?

Would the governments agree to create an independent body to investigate and test, because I am sure that the evolution of many diseases is not trivial in our cities.

Beyond drugs, I have also always been concerned about the toxicity of the chemical molecules that surround us: those that we see but also those that cannot be seen but are breathed in. The number of cancers is exploding.Many sick and dead people are already due to pollution! 9 million deaths per year in the world, it is enormous but how many more are due to the invisible pollution of all these substances of which we do not speak.

In the meantime, journalists are aware that they have a mission in this field, to make things move forward by making official the information which, for the moment, only circulates discreetly among informed people. We would have thought that with the Internet everything would go faster but it is always too slow.

The success of organic food shows that mentalities are changing and that risk prevention is important for many people, but how many continue to consume non-organic food? Do we really have to make a choice between vegetables contaminated by insecticides and those that are not, or should these contaminated vegetables and fruits not even be sold? Do we have to choose between an expensive, non-toxic product and a cheap, toxic one? And here I come to the heart of the subject of this book: an "E" that punctuates the composition of consumer products and medicines.

The use of food codes (E...) prevents us from seeing the chemical name of the ingredients of the substances we ingest. It would surely be less appetizing and especially less selling! How much time do we spend checking the components of our food during our shopping? Do we really know what we are eating and absorbing? Why not imagine, for example, a color code to identify toxic products directly on the products?

Isn't the communication around obesity responsible for this excessive presence of aspartame in our food? "Sugar is bad! Long live aspartame!" But we do not talk about aspartame, we say *light*, it gives a certain legitimacy. Is this part of the marketing strategy of the products and their success? We often talk about the precautionary principle but what about aspartame? Many studies are conducted but the results are often contradictory. Some claim to reveal a terrible toxicity, others a relative toxicity. Should we wait until we officially discover that aspartame is really dangerous, just like similar molecules, before reacting and banning it, or should we mention the risks linked to its consumption, or should we assume that as long as this has not been demonstrated, we can consume it without reservation?

We are pleased to see the "danger/pregnancy" logo appear on drugs that contain active ingredients that are dangerous during pregnancy, but we can deplore the fact that there is no logo if this danger can come from the excipients.

Sugar-free" in pharmacies is legitimate to take into account pathologies that do not allow its consumption, but should we be forced to take aspartame? These excipients that are supposed to be without consequences are far from being so, especially when we measure, for example, the catastrophic consequences on thousands of patients caused by the change of excipient in levothyrox.It was supposed to be an improvement... Many nicotine substitutes are consumed daily and contain aspartame.Is this the price to pay to stop smoking?Is this the only solution?

At the counter, it is often the example of aspartame that I use with my clients to illustrate the risks of using expired products. Indeed, aspartame is fragile, unstable over time, and chemically modifies itself to become a mutagenic molecule; this also allows us to better understand the short expiration dates of sodas that contain it.

Aspartame is present in many beverages, but although very unstable above 30°C, it can be found in many hot countries or even, during the summer in France, stored at much higher temperatures for weeks without any control or conservation precautions on the product, but what a joy to sip a well iced soda in the sun!

Will you still do it after reading this book?

Franck Cohen, Doctor of Pharmacy, graduate of Paris XI

Appendix 2 - Official FDA text

Code of Federal Regulations]
[Title 21, Volume 3]
[Revised as of April 1, 2014]
[CITE: 21CFR172.804]
TITLE 21--FOOD AND DRUGS
CHAPTER I--FOOD AND DRUG ADMINISTRATION
DEPARTMENT OF HEALTH AND HUMAN SERVICES
SUBCHAPTER B--FOOD FOR HUMAN CONSUMPTION
(CONTINUED)

PART 172--FOOD ADDITIVES PERMITTED FOR DIRECT ADDITION TO FOOD FOR HUMAN CONSUMPTION
Subpart I--Multipurpose Additives
Sec. 172.804 Aspartame.

The food additive aspartame may be safely used in food in accordance with good manufacturing practice as a sweetening agent and a flavor enhancer in foods for which standards of identity established under section 401 of the act do not preclude such use under the following conditions:

(a) Aspartame is the chemical 1-methyl N- l- [alpha]-aspartyl-l-phenylalanine (C14H18N2O5).

(b) The additive meets the specifications of the Food Chemicals Codex, 7th ed. (2010), pp. 73-74, which is incorporated by reference. The Director of the Office of the Federal Register approves this incorporation by reference in accordance with 5 U.S.C. 552 (a) and 1 CFR part 51. You may obtain copies from the United States

Pharmacopeial Convention, 12601 Twinbrook Pkwy., Rockville, MD 20852 (Internet address usp.org). Copies may be examined at the Food and Drug Administration's Main Library, 10903 New Hampshire Ave, Bldg. 2, Third Floor, Silver Spring, MD 20993, 301-796-2039, or at the National Archives and Records Administration (NARA). For information on the availability of this material at NARA, call 202-741-6030 or go to archives.gov/federal-register...

(c) (1) When aspartame is used as a sugar substitute tablet for sweetening hot beverages, including coffee and tea, L-leucine may be used as a lubricant in the manufacture of such tablets at a level not to exceed 3.5 percent of the weight of the tablet.

(2) When aspartame is used in baked goods and baking mixes, the amount of the additive is not to exceed 0.5 percent by weight of ready-to-bake products or of finished formulations prior to baking. Generally recognized as safe (GRAS) ingredients or food additives approved for use in baked goods shall be used in combination with aspartame to ensure its functionality as a sweetener in the final baked product. The level of aspartame used in these products is determined by an analytical method entitled "Analytical Method for the Determination of Aspartame and Diketopiperazine in Baked Goods and Baking Mixes," October 8, 1992, which was developed by the Nutrasweet Co. Copies are available from the Office of Premarket Approval (HFS-200), Center for Food Safety and Applied Nutrition, 5100 Paint Branch Pkwy., College Park, MD 20740, or are available for inspection at the Center for Food Safety and Applied Nutrition's Library, Food and Drug Administration, 5100 Paint Branch Pkwy., College Park, MD 20740, and at the National Archives and Records Administration (NARA). For information on the availability of this material at NARA, call 202-741-6030, or go to: archives.gov/federal.../...

(d) To assure safe use of the additive, in addition to the other information required by the Act :

(1) The principal display panel of any intermediate mix of the additive for manufacturing purposes shall bear a statement of the concentration of the additive contained therein ;

(2) The label of any food containing the additive shall bear, either on the principal display panel or on the information panel, the following statement:

PHENYLKETONURICS : CONTAINS PHENYLALANINE
The statement shall appear in the labeling prominently and conspicuously as compared to other words, statements, designs or devices and in bold type and on clear contrasting background in order to render it likely to be read and understood by the ordinary individual under customary conditions of purchase and use.

(3) When the additive is used in a sugar substitute for table use, its label shall bear instructions not to use in cooking or baking.

(4) Packages of the dry, free-flowing additive shall prominently display the sweetening equivalence in teaspoons of sugar.

(e) If the food containing the additive purports to be or is represented for special dietary uses, it shall be labeled in compliance with part 105 of this chapter.

[39 FR 27319, July 26, 1974]

Editorial Note:
For Federal Register citations affecting 172.804, see the List of CFR Sections Affected, which appears in the Finding Aids section of the printed volume and at government Publishing Office. (www. fdsys.gov.)

APPENDIX 3

Dear Jeffrey,

I have a question that really needs answering. How can aspartame be considered safe when independent scientific research consistently shows that it can be deadly? Has EFSA decided to ignore all the damning research and only accept the studies funded by the aspartame industry? Example: EFSA uses the Ajinomoto study - funded by the industry and its conflicts of interest, and ignores the huge contradiction of scientific research.

To help EFSA understand the industry's cover-up methods, researcher Mark Gold has scrupulously detailed their scientific abuses in the aspartame studies.

There is abundant evidence of scientific abuse in studies of the effects of aspartame on Parkinson's disease, methanol toxicity, etc. A government agency that must be impartial, must avoid conflicts of interest and consider only scientific research published by independent journals and qualified experts around the world. These consistently show that aspartame is deadly. EFSA's modus operandi is to ignore this real science. What a shame!

It was the Parliament that asked for a new evaluation because they saw that research showed that aspartame was dangerous (study in Denmark on 60,000 women showing that aspartame causes a jump in premature births, up to 78%, and the three studies of Dr. Morando Soffritti, of the Ramazzini Institute showing that aspartame is a multipotential carcinogen) causing lung and liver cancers as well as leukemia and breast cancer.

Another list outlines research on kidney destruction, heart attacks and strokes caused by soda consumption.

Egyptian research has revealed destructive effects on memory and oxidative stress in the brains of mice, and its study shows that aspartame increases fasting blood sugar, and a study shows that aspartame can cause severe depression.

A Harvard study proved that aspartame can cause Hodgkin's lymphoma and leukemia, confirming the work of Dr. Soffritti.

Another study links aspartame to diabetes, as has been known for thirty years. Endocrinologist H. J. Roberts says that aspartame not only precipitates diabetes, but aggravates and simulates diabetic retinopathy and neuropathy; methanol conversion destroys the optic nerve and causes seizures. It even interacts with insulin. These are recent studies!

You realize that I could go on and on about the scientific research that proves over and over again that aspartame is deadly. You are well aware of Trocho's study[110] which showed that aspartame embalms living tissue and degrades DNA.

Read the last chapter of While Science Sleeps by Dr. Woodrow Monte.

This shows beyond a shadow of a doubt that the FDA knew that aspartame caused birth defects before it was approved, this having been negotiated with the manufacturer to seal the studies and never allow the public to know the truth. It produces autism epidemics! In the United States 1 in 50 school children is autistic[111].

Even Dr. Herman Koëter[112] who headed the EFSA scientific committee has admitted to being pushed by industry to hijack the science.

Just one of these studies could get aspartame banned, but there are so many! EFSA uses rigged industry research to refute/ignore legitimate and honest studies. If 100 unbiased researchers studying aspartame prove

---

110. Extract from an article in *France-Soir*, April 1st, 2009: "In 1998, a Spanish study conducted by Dr. Carme Trocho (Faculty of Biology at the University of Barcelona) concluded that DNA was damaged by an accumulation of formaldehyde in organs, particularly the brain, in vitro. It remained to prove the carcinogenic character in vivo. This was done last May by the Ramazzini Institute.

111. In any case, the number of children diagnosed has risen sharply: between 2006 and 2008, the number of children diagnosed has increased by more than 20%. One child out of 88 was affected in 2008. The evolution is all the more significant as only 1 child out of 110 had received the same diagnosis in 2006. These figures are from 2012 for 14-state studies of 8-year-olds. Boys are five times more affected than girls. In France, there is 1 child with autism out of 100.

112. Dr. Koëter is a toxicologist and nutrition specialist.

that it is dangerous, will EFSA ignore and refute them all as it has done in the past? EFSA's history provides the answer.

So my initial question is why does EFSA approve aspartame when almost all independent studies show it to be very harmful? When I say almost all independent studies, you should take into account Dr. Ralph Walton's research: he found that 92% of all independent studies showed that aspartame was not safe. However, he also said that if you eliminate the six FDA studies that were controversial because they were linked to the food industry, 100% found aspartame unsafe. To date, we have exposed industry studies that try to show safety, when in fact they show scientific abuse. You can't take a chemical poison and show it's safe. Even FDA toxicologist Dr. Jacqueline Verrett said in 1987 that aspartame had not yet been proven safe, and that was six years after it was approved.

In fact, the FDA's senior toxicologist, Dr. Adrian Gross, told Congress that aspartame violated the Delaney Amendment because of brain tumors and brain cancer. The Delaney Amendment prohibits adding anything to food and drugs that can cause cancer. He also stated that the FDA would not have been able to define a tolerable daily intake, and if the FDA violated its own laws, what is left to protect the public? Because he kept talking about aspartame, he was fired from the EPA (Environmental Protection Agency)! You also know that aspartame was approved in England thanks to a business agreement between G.D. Searle and Paul Turner. No studies have been done in the UK.

Without a doubt, EFSA is not protecting Europeans, as it has an innate conflict of interest due to its loyalty to the manufacturers/distributors of aspartame. To hell with the people of Europe! Let them die.

I know Jeff, that you can't be on this committee anymore, but you know where to send this for a response. I have some names. Make sure you read this.

Following is a list of sites given by Dr. Betty Martini: to be found on her site on scientific abuses and possible fraud in the research on Monsanto's aspartame, in the research on migraine and link with the Dorway site.

APPENDIX 4 - *WALL STREET JOURNAL*, FEBRUARY 7, 1986

It is learned that two former prosecutors investigating Searle were interviewed as witnesses by Andy Pasztor and Joe Davidson in Washington, D.C. They are two government attorneys who are determined to attack the maker of NutraSweet, accused of falsifying test results during the criminal and senatorial investigations. The documents shown yesterday by Senator Howard Metzenbaum (Ohio) are the fruits of the investigation by Samuel Skinner and William Conlon, two senior prosecutors from the Chicago Department of Justice against G. D. Searle & Co. and repeated requests via the Food and Drug Administration. There was material to submit to the grand jury during the 1970s. The documents prove that the two key figures Skinner and Conlon later joined Sidley & Austin, a firm that was already representing Searle throughout the criminal investigation. In April 1976, the documents show that the FDA was pressing Justice to form a grand jury to determine whether Searle had allowed documents to be truncated before they were turned over to the government. In January 1977, the FDA urgently requested a thorough investigation of NutraSweet, the most popular sweetener, and also of Aldactone, a blood pressure product. Richard Merrill, then FDA Chief Counsel, sent a 33-page report to Skinner that included details about "FALSE SPECIFIC STATEMENTS AND DISSIMULATIONS OF ACTS" regarding internal testing of Searle's own aspartame, now sold as NutraSweet. The report urgently called for a grand jury investigation into the company for "WILLFUL FAILURE TO COMPLY", which had gutted the report by "DISSIMULATION OF MATERIAL EVIDENCE". The Grand Jury investigation was launched in August, but only the hypertension drug was investigated, the other subject being shelved, without any prosecution until 1979. Senator Metzenbaum applied his research to the whole chain, and it was then that serious questions arose about the "aggressiveness" of Justice. He called for a full investigation into whether the first two prosecutors had done wrong and why... The senator repeated his criticism of Justice for failing to prosecute white collar crime. According to Metzenbaum, it was vital that the harmfulness of artificial sugar was finally and independently investigated. A speaker from the FDA said that there was no new scientific information in the requested report, which meant that the producers had a free hand. The senators' investigation stated that Searle was located in Skokie, a suburb of Chicago, Illinois, and that a Monsanto Co. unit was located in St. Louis, and that previously untraceable answers would be revealed. That's what the senator says. His assertions point to serious lapses. In a statement, Skinner said he quickly withdrew from any involvement after receiving an official letter from the FDA in his office requesting a grand jury. He stood by his statement about conflicts of interest. Mr. Conlon did not return phone calls. In a March 1977 memo, Skinner, then Chicago's attorney general, told other Justice Department lawyers that he was withdrawing from any involvement in the Searle investigation. He asked his subordinates to keep this confidential from law enforcement officials to avoid embarrassment. Senator Metzenbaum wanted to determine whether Skinner was discussing the job with Sidley & Austin before he moved on, or whether he had already been greased? Skinner's successor took his place months later when the lawsuit had expired. Federal conflicts of interest generally prohibit government officials from getting involved in private matters to discuss hiring for a position... Those in the Washington Justice Department complained in April and August 1977 about delays in responding to the grand jury. In October 1977, Conlon, the Chief Prosecutor, under too much work and pressure, showed redacted documents. The case was closed. Skinner joined Sidley & Austin in July 1977, Conlon waited to join the firm in January 1979. At that time, the judge notified the FDA that the case was closed...

APPENDIX 5

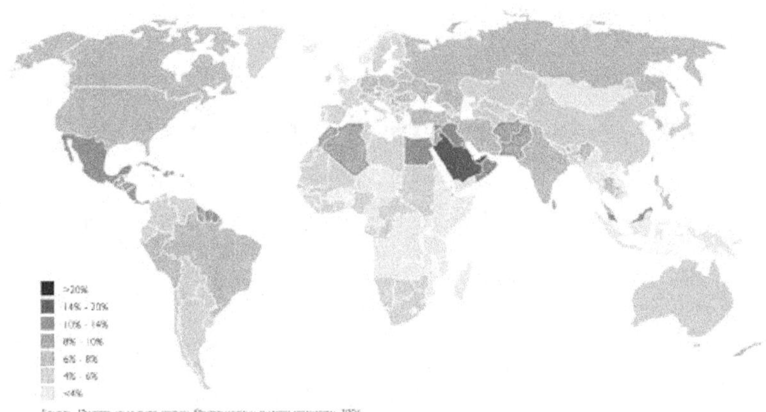

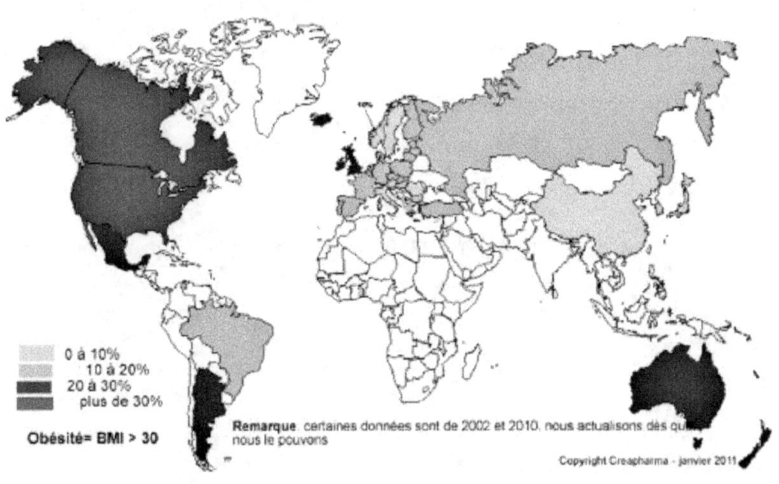

Appendix 5

HAUSSE DU DIABÈTE DE TYPE 2 DEPUIS 1980

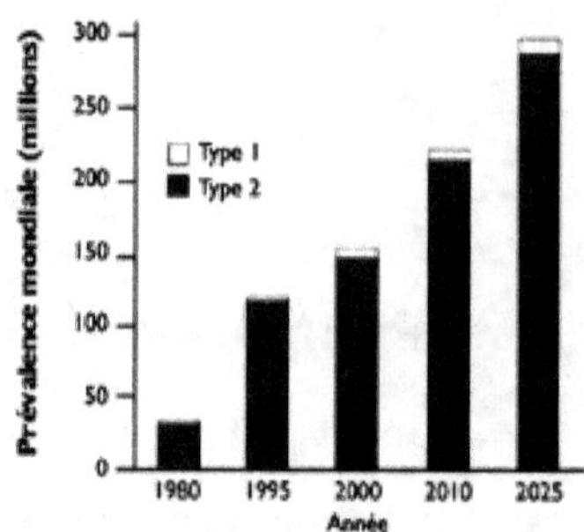

L'OBÈSITÉ EN POURCENTAGES DE POPULATION

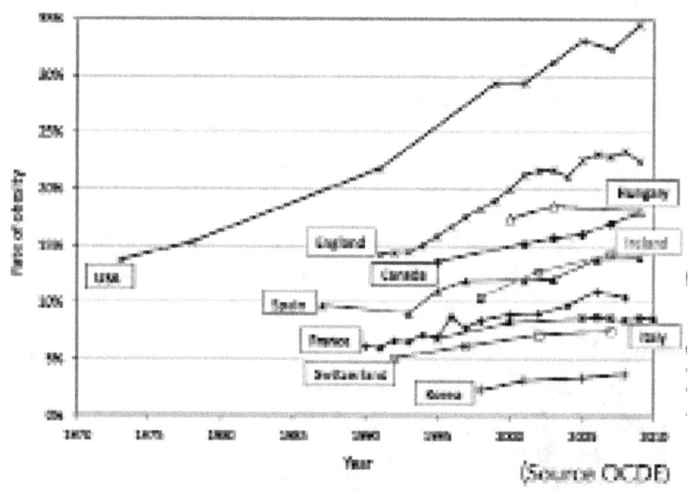

On this map, obesity in percentages of the population

APPENDIX 6

Les cas de démence devraient tripler d'ici 2050
La démence, notamment la maladie d'Alzheimer, un des plus gros défis de santé publique
En millions de cas, par région
2013 2030 2050
Prévisions
71,8
20,8
14,8
10,9
Europe
39,8
30,5
21,9
15,8
8,8
Amériques
12,4
6,2
2,8
Afrique
Asie-Pacifique
135
Estimations révisées
Premières estimations
115
Cas de démence dans le monde
(en millions)
76
44
65
36
2010   2013   2030   2050
Source :
Alzheimer's Disease International
AFP

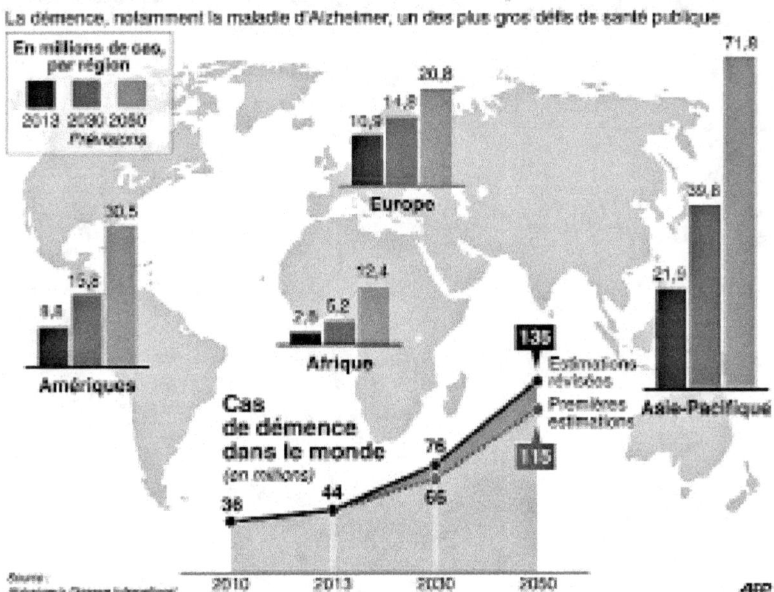

The growing cost of Alzheimer's Disease

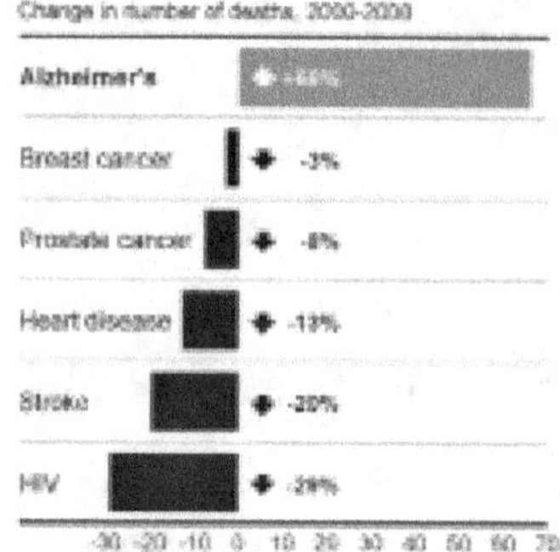

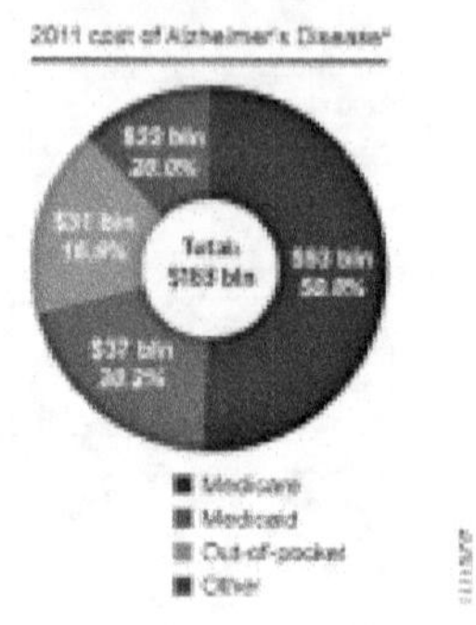

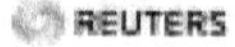

* Percentages may not total 100 due to rounding
Source: Alzheimer's Association

REUTERS

Appendix 7 - Some excerpts on the proposed "Aspartame Tax"

"Art. I. - It is instituted a special tax on aspartame, coded E951 in the European classification of food additives, actually intended, as is or after incorporation into all products, for human consumption.

"II. - The rate of the additional tax is set per kilogram at €30 in 2013, €50 in 2014, €70 in 2015 and €90 from 2016. This rate is increased on January 1 of each year starting January 1, 2017. To this end, the rate of the tax is revised each year in December, by order of the minister in charge of the budget published in the Official Journal, according to the forecasted annual average change for the following year in consumer prices for all households excluding tobacco prices. The forecasted changes taken into account are those appearing in the economic, social and financial report appended to the last finance bill.

"III. - 1. The contribution is due on account of food aspartame or food products incorporating it by their manufacturers established in France, their importers and persons who make intra-Community acquisitions in France, on all quantities delivered or incorporated for valuable consideration or free of charge.

" 2. Are also liable for the contribution the persons who, within the framework of their commercial activity, incorporate, for the products intended for the food of their customers, of the aspartame.

"IV. - For food products, taxation is carried out according to the quantity of aspartame entering their composition.

"V. - Aspartame or food products incorporating it exported from mainland France and Corsica, which are the subject of a delivery exempted under I of Article 262 ter or a delivery to a place located in another Member State of the European Union pursuant to Article 258 A, are not subject to the special tax.

"VI. - The special tax shall be established and collected in accordance with the procedures and under the securities, guarantees and penalties applicable to turnover taxes.

"However, the special measures and accounting requirements necessary to ensure that the special tax is levied only on aspartame actually intended for human consumption, that it is collected only once, and that it is not borne in the event of export, delivery exempted under Article 262 ter or delivery to a place located in another Member State of the European Union pursuant to Article 258 A, shall be determined by decree.

"VII. - The proceeds of this tax shall be allocated to the fund mentioned in Article L. 135-1 of the Social Security Code."

Object

Present in thousands of everyday food products, aspartame is the most widely used intense sweetener in the world. As soon as it appeared in the 1960s in the United States, doubts arose about its harmfulness and its marketing was immediately marred by conflicts of interest. In 1985, the firm Monsanto bought the company that owned the patent.

For pregnant women, studies have shown that, even at low doses, aspartame increases the risk of preterm birth. In addition, there are very strong presumptions that the consumption of aspartame leads to an increased risk of various cancers.

This amendment creates an additional tax on aspartame, scheduled to increase each year until 2016. Indeed, the first objective is to encourage manufacturers to substitute aspartame with other sweeteners, natural or synthetic. To this end, it is necessary to remove its competitive advantage, which is based solely on the fact that the cost of health damage it causes is externalized and borne by the community. From this point of view, progressivity is essential because it allows to reach a dissuasive taxation in the long term while leaving the industrialists time to adapt to the substitute products. Imports are obviously also taxed.

The annual consumption in France is estimated at about 1500 tons. The revenue from the tax would therefore be 45 million in 2013; 75 million in 2014; 105 million in 2015; 135 million per year from 2016. At that point, we will be able to judge whether or not it is appropriate to extend the increase.

For a box of 300 candy bars with a weight of 15g, the extra cost is 50 cents in 2013, 80 cents in 2014, 1.10 euros in 2015 and 1.40 euros from 2016.

Obviously, the substitution of aspartame by other products will reduce the base and therefore the yield of the tax. Until substitution takes place, the revenue generated will be used to finance prevention policies.

Taxation is preferred to prohibition because, except in the case of pregnant women, it has not yet been demonstrated that consumption at low doses is harmful. For pregnant women, the authors propose in another amendment to add a health warning on the packaging of products containing aspartame. In addition, the authors consider that it is urgent to conduct independent studies on the health risks associated with the consumption of aspartame. The proceeds of this tax could be used to finance them.

Because the creation of a prevention fund by amendment is prohibited by Article 40 of the Constitution, this amendment appropriates the revenue from this tax to Medicare."

From the moments of the session we can retain the speech of Aline Archimbaud, a senator who is not afraid of lobbies:

Sweetened beverages, an important source of profit for the food industry, are the nightmare of nutritionists. Among many studies in the same direction, the one conducted in 2010 by Professor Frank Hu, from the Harvard School of Public Health, in Boston, showed that there was a link between excess consumption of sweetened beverages and obesity, but also the occurrence of type 2 diabetes and cardiovascular diseases. In France, nearly 15% of adults are now affected by obesity, which represents an increase of more than 10% since 2006. We are indeed dealing with a pandemic, i.e. the rapid increase in the incidence of a disease present over a large geographical area. Obesity has become the fifth leading cause of death in the world, even catching up with the number of deaths due

Appendix 7 - Some excerpts on the proposed "Aspartame Tax"

to smoking in the United States. Obese people are more susceptible to heart disease and stroke, diabetes, degenerative diseases, breast and colon cancer. The costs to our social protection system are in the billions of euros. To give you an example, the French association of diabetics, which counts three million people suffering from this pathology, estimates that diabetes alone costs the social security system more than 17 billion euros each year. This figure, given very recently, is higher than the deficit noted each year in the execution of the social security financing laws!

The situation is far too serious for us to stand idly by as this scourge spreads. This amendment therefore aims to double the tax on sugary drinks in order to limit their consumption. It also aims to double the tax on drinks containing aspartame, in order to avoid making them relatively cheaper, which would encourage their consumption and would be in total contradiction with the amendment I will present to you later on this sweetener.

Jacques Mézard also wanted to amend the tax on sodas and other sugary drinks by 50%. He added:

Indeed, we consider that these drinks contribute to the prevalence of obesity and are certainly one of the factors that explain the considerable increase in diabetes. The risk is particularly significant for children, for whom the consumption of sweetened beverages is, in general, considered very worrying by many doctors. It is true that we do not have enough time to assess the impact of the tax that has been in place for less than a year. Nevertheless, we consider that our proposal is consistent with all the measures defended by the government in this bill. It is a public health measure, a behavioral signal, as for tobacco or beer. In any case, Madam Minister, it will be necessary to evaluate all these behavioral taxes in the framework of the public health bill that you will present to us."
What was the opinion of the Government that the president asked Mrs. Marisol Touraine, Minister of Social Affairs and Health? *The Government has the same opinion as the Commission, Mr. Chairman, and for the same reasons. "I would like to remind you that the existing tax was introduced a short time ago and that we do not have sufficient hindsight to assess its effect on consumption. It is on the basis of such an evaluation that we will be able to put in place long-term strategies*

within the framework of the future public health law. Furthermore, and I will no doubt have the opportunity to repeat this during the rest of the discussion, I am not sure that it is good policy to multiply contributions or taxes on food products without considering globally how this fits in with a public health policy on the one hand, and with the financing of social protection on the other.../...This is why I am asking for the withdrawal of these amendments, which will otherwise be rejected. The risk would be to find ourselves without a clear vision of how these taxes can have a long-term impact on the financing of social security and on consumer behavior. Whatever one's opinion of the products in question - and I don't think anyone would argue that abusing soft drinks or sugary drinks is good for one's health - it seems preferable to be able to assess the impact of the tax that has already been passed.

BIBLIOGRAPHY

BAUER Werner J., BADOUD Raphaël, LÖLIGER Jürg, ETOURNAUD Alain: *Science et technologie des aliments. Principes de chimie des constituants et de technologie des procédés*, Presses polytechniques et universitaires romandes, Lausanne, 2010.

BLAYLOCK Russel L.: *Excitotoxins, The Taste that Kills*, Health Press, Santa Fe (NM, USA), 1997.

BRANEN A. Larry, DAVIDSON R. Michael, SALMINEN Seppo, THORNGATE III John H.: *Food Additives*, Marcel Dekker, Inc., New York, NW, USA and Basel, Switzerland, second revised and expanded edition, 2002.

COCKBRURN Andrew: *Rumsfeld : His rise, Fall, and Catastrophic Legacy*, Simon and Schuster, New York (NW, USA), 2007.

DAVIS Devra: *The Secret History of the War of Cancer*, Basic Books, New York, NW, USA, 2007.

DIEMER Tom: *Fighting the Unbeatable Foe: Howard Metzenbaum of Ohio, the Washington Years*, The Kent State University Press, Kent, OH, USA, 2008.

EVANGELISTA Arthur M.: "Aspartame: The History Of A Killer - The Whole Story", URL http://www.rense.com/general50/killer.htm

FILER JR. L. J. and STEGINK Lewis D.: "Aspartame: Physiology and Biochemistry" *in* Pieter WALSTRA (ed.), *Physical Chemistry of Foods*, Marcel Dekker, Inc., New York, NY, USA, 2003.

GILLESPIE David: *Sweet Poison, Why Sugar make Us Fat*, Penguin Group USA, New York, NW, USA, 2013.

GOLD Mark D.: "The Bitter Truth About Artificial Sweetener", *Nexus Magazine*, Vol. 2, October-November 1995 and Vol. 3, December 1995-January 1996.

JY Kim, SEO J., KH Cho: "Aspartame-fed zebrafish exhibit acute deaths with swimming defects and saccharin-fed zebrafish have elevation of cholesteryl ester transfer protein activity in hypercholesterolemia", *Food Chem Toxicol*, 2011, vol. 49, p. 2899-2905.

MARTIN Hans-Peter and SCHUMANN Harald: *Le Piège de la mondialisation*, Solin-Actes Sud, Arles and Paris, 1997.

MONTE Woodrow C.: *While Science Sleeps: A Sweetener Kills*, Amazon Create Space Publishing, San Francisco, CA, USA, 2011.

NASH STODDARD Mary: *Deadly Deception: Story of Aspartame: Shocking Expose of the World's Most Controversial Sweetener*, Odenwald Press, Dallas, Tx, USA, 1998.

OLNEY JW: "Brain lesions, obesity, and other disturbances in mice treated with monosodium glutamate", *Science*, No. 164, May 9, 1969, pp. 719-721.

OM Abdel-Salam, NA Salem, HUSSEIN Jihan Seid: "Effect of Aspartame on Oxidative Stress and Monoamine Neurotransmitter Levels in Lipopolysaccharide-Treated Mice", *Neurotox Res.,21*, pp. 245-255, 2011 Aug. 6. Department of Toxicology and Narcotics, National Research Centre, Tahrir St., Dokki, Cairo (Egypt), 2011.

POTHUIZEN Helen HJ, JONGEN-RÊLO Ana L., FELDON Joram: "Preclinical Research: The Effects of Temporary Inactivation of the Core and the Shell Subregions of the Nucleus Accumbens on Prepulse Inhibition of the Acoustic Startle Reflex and Activity in Rats," Department of pharmacology, Chicago Ill., USA, 2005.

PRYER Douglas A. (Major): *The Fight For The High Ground: The U.S. Army And Interrogation During Operation Iraqi Freedom I, May 2003-April 2004*, Pickle Partners Publishing, Overdrive, Inc., Cleveland Ohio, USA, 2015.

RADMAN Miroslav et CARTON Daniel: *Au delà de nos limites biologiques*, Plon, Paris, 2011.

ROBERTS H.J.: *Aspartame (NutraSweet) Is It Safe?* Charles Press, Philadelphia. 1990, and *Aspartame Disease, an ignored epidemic*, Sunshine sentinel Press. Inc, West Palm Beach, Fla., USA, 2001.

STARR HULL Janet S.: *Sweet Poison: How the World's Most Popular Artificial Sweetener Is Killing Us – My Story*, New Horizon Press, Far Hills, NJ, USA, 1998.

STEINERT R., FREY F., TÖPFER A., DREWE J., BERLINGER C.: "Effects of carbohydrate sugars and artificial sweeteners on appetite and the secretion of gastrointestinal satiety peptides", *Br J Nutr.*, 2011, Division of Gastroenterology, Department of Biomedicine, Clinical Research Center, University Hospital Basel, Basel, Switzerland.

TURNER James S., NADER Ralph: *The Chemical Feast, The Ralph Nader Study Group Report on Food Protection and the Food and Drug Administration*, Penguin Books USA, New York, NY, USA, 1976.

VERRETT Jacqueline et CARPER Jean: *Eating May Be Hazardous to Your Health*, Anchor Press/ Doubleday, Garden City, NY, USA, 1975.

WAISMAN Harry: *Disorders of Amino Acid Metabolism and Mental Retardation*, Spinger 1995.

See also the videos on edu/news

Other

Interviews and conferences :

BLAYLOCK Russell L., interview by Mike Adams (Septembre 27, 2006), on naturalnews.com/

BRESSLER Jerome: History of the U.S. Food and Drug Administration: interview by Robert A. Tucker, on doorway.com

See also the Diet Pepsi for a new generation clips on YouTube.

MAGNUSON lecture: What Health Professionals Need to Know About Aspartame From Metabolism and Safety to Impact on Appetite and Body Weight. See the site where Ms. Magnuson explains the non-toxicity for pregnant women and babies: on her site and others.

Table of Contents

BEST SELLERS MAX MILO EDITIONS

Hitler's banker, Jean-François Bouchard

Confessions of a forger, Éric Piedoie Le Tiec

The Koran and the flesh, Ludovic-Mohamed Zahed

Governing by fake news, Jacques Baud

Governing by chaos, Collectif

A political history of food, Paul Ariès

Mad in U.S.A.: The ravages of the "American model",
Michel Desmurget

Mondial soccer club geopolitics, Kévin Veyssière

Putin: Game master?, Jacques Braud

Treatise on the three impostors: Moses, Jesus, Muhammad,
The Spirit of Spinoza

TV Lobotomy, Michel Desmurget

www.ingramcontent.com/pod-product-compliance
Lightning Source LLC
LaVergne TN
LVHW050419060726
842526LV00008B/2683